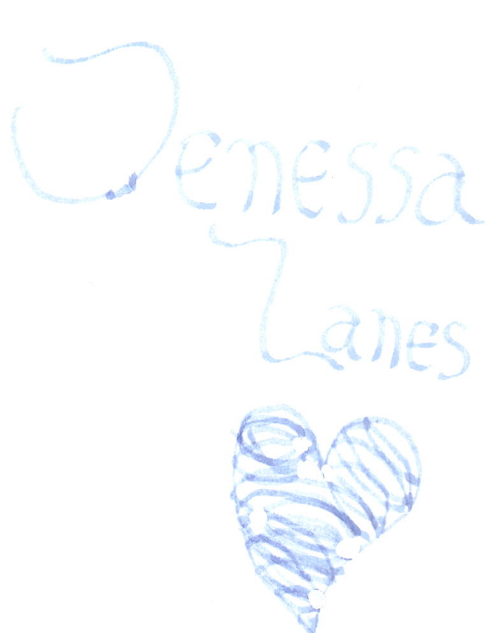
Jenessa
Lanes

WHAT BLIND PEOPLE WISH SIGHTED PEOPLE KNEW ABOUT BLINDNESS!

by Harry Martin

Revised Edition
Harry Martin Publishing
Orlando, Florida, USA
407-207-4777

WHAT BLIND PEOPLE WISH SIGHTED PEOPLE KNEW ABOUT BLINDNESS!

Many letters received were generalized and names were not used to protect the privacy of the writers. Where contributors authorized the use of their name letters were used as quotations, and the author included their names.

Printed in the United States of America
by Harry Martin Publishing.

First Printing - 1996
Second Printing - 1997
Revised Edition - 1997
ISBN 0-9652205-0-8

DEDICATION

This book is lovingly dedicated to my wife,
Carol,
whose constant love and support
helped make this book possible.

And to the memory of my nephew,
Christopher Michael Martin,
who is deeply missed and fondly
remembered.

TABLE OF CONTENTS:

ACKNOWLEDGMENT

I want to take this opportunity to give special acknowledgment to my wife, Carol, for proofreading the manuscript of this book. Carol is a home health care nurse and works extremely hard caring for her patients. I know it was not easy for her to take what little spare time she had to read the manuscript to my book and give me her critique on it.

I also want to thank her for allowing me to relate our own experiences to the reader in the chapter entitled, "TIPS ON BEING A SIGHTED SPOUSE." It is not easy to let your husband write about one's own problems in a book that is going to get read by the public. Her being willing to let me share our experience will, we both hope, help other married couples deal with problems that occur due to one of them being blind.

I wish everyone could be blest with a loving, dedicated wife like Carol. She is a true friend, and I love her.

INTRODUCTION

I spent a number of years going blind as the result of a service connected disability. My blindness began as a mild visual impairment in 1973, during a stint in the Navy. It grew worse over twenty-three years until I was blind in both eyes. My left eye was removed due to extreme pain from glaucoma in 1993. This progression from being fully sighted to being blind allowed me to experience the full range of frustrations, emotions, problems, and attitudes that all blind and visually impaired people encounter. As someone who experiences blindness on a daily basis, who experienced going blind over a long period, I feel I am qualified to write a book about what blind people go through, how they feel, and what they wish sighted people knew about the blind.

I was led to write this book by my fellow blind friends who felt there was a lot about blind people that sighted people did not understand. While there was already a large selection of books about blindness and blind people, many were not available to the sighted public at large. Many were written in such a technical manner they would not appeal to the public. My blind friends felt that despite the many existing books about blindness, there was room for another book. A book written with a positive tone to help educate the sighted public about what it is like to be blind in a sighted world. Most important, that it be a book written by a blind person who knew from experience about the subject, blindness.

In writing this book, I have attempted to stay away from the technical explanations of blindness when possible. Explaining the different levels of blindness in Chapter One was necessary to help sighted readers understand how a person can be blind and still see something. Or, why one blind person's condition can be so different from another. Apart from this brief explanation of blindness, I wanted to deal with the human side of being blind in a sighted world.

I also tried to find out what blind people, as a group, felt sighted people should know about blind people and being blind. I did not want to presume to know how all blind people felt about living in a sighted world. So, I invited blind people all over the United States and Canada to write to me and tell me what they thought sighted people should know about blindness. Because of this invitation, I heard from hundreds of blind people who did, in fact, have some things they wanted sighted people to know about their blindness. They were things that had not been dealt with in other books they had read about blindness and the blind, or that was not covered from their perspective. Much of what my blind friends had to say to sighted people found its way into this book.

The reader should also understand when they read this book, it is the voices of hundreds of blind people speaking out to help educate their sighted friends on what it is like to be blind in a sighted world. This book is not something I just sat down one day and decided to write based only on my own experiences or opinions. However, I have used a number of my own experiences, along with those of the blind people who responded to my request for their ideas. I felt if I were going to relate the experiences of other blind people who cared enough to share their experiences, I should be willing to share some of my own. I do know that my experiences have been shared by hundreds of other blind men and women, just as I have shared many experiences they related to me, some of which appear in this book.

There is also a chapter in this book about what blind

people wish other blind people knew about blindness. As I conducted my research for this book, I heard from a number of blind people who felt that many blind people do not understand each other. I can say from experience that this is sometimes true. Because our conditions and agendas can be so different, it is common to find blind people who are misinformed about each others conditions and capabilities. All blind people have encountered blind colleagues who feel it is their calling to tell all other blind people how to dress, eat, think or what mobility aids they should, or should not use. So, I have attempted to deal with that matter in this book. If the blind cannot deal with their own misinformation and shortcomings, we cannot ask our sighted friends to deal with theirs.

I also want to emphasize that this book is not a forum for whining blind people. None of the blind people who contributed their thoughts to this book wrote to me with that attitude. All the letters were written in a positive tone; and the writers all wished to help promote a better understanding between the blind and the sighted. I suspect the whiners just never bothered contributing at all. The sighted reader should read this book with the understanding I mean this book as an informative educational tool to help them better understand and relate to their blind friends, coworkers, spouses, or relatives. If there are portions of this book that sound like whining, I would say that it was necessary to be honest on some of the problems with which the blind have to deal. Such sections, as blunt as they may be, are meant to produce a positive understanding in the way sighted people deal with the blind, or how blind people deal with each other.

What I hope this book accomplishes is this. I hope the sighted people who read it go away with a better understanding of how to deal with and treat blind people they encounter in public, or with blind friends or family members. I hope that the blind people who read this book also gain a better understanding of the fact that not all blind people are alike in terms of coping skills, or in dealing with their blindness.

One thing is certain; despite all the books on the market, there is an amazing lack of understanding in the community about blindness. Every day, I encounter people, both blind and sighted, who do not know what it is like to be blind. If some of the sighted people I have encountered just knew a little bit more about blindness, my day might have gone better. As amazing as it may sound, there are many days I find that if some blind people knew more about blindness, both their day ***and*** my day might have gone better. If this is true in my case, I know it is true for thousands of other blind people as well.

The last thing I want to say in this Introduction is this. This book does not have any agenda. It does not promote braille over recorded books, or, cane use over guide dogs. It does not advocate membership in any specific blind organizations or political action groups. I do not intend this book to further any cause, other than to promote a better understanding about what blindness is and how to deal with blind people better. If I have accomplished that goal, then this book was more than worth the effort required to bring it to the public. I may not win any awards for writing style, or championing a specific cause. However, if sighted people can read this book and look on blindness, and the blind, in a more positive light, I will be satisfied.

WHY CAN SOME BLIND PEOPLE SEE?

The most common misconception I have encountered as a blind person is all blind people are totally blind. This was the subject of many letters I received from blind people in response to my invitation to contribute their ideas. Yet, according to the American Foundation for the Blind, only 4% of all blind people are totally blind. What that means is that the vast majority of blind people ***see*** something. This confuses not only many sighted people, but many blind people and service providers as well.

Blindness is just like any other disability. It afflicts people in varying degrees. The fact that one person is afflicted more severely than another does not make the other person any less afflicted. A person who is paralyzed from the waist down is paralyzed. A person paralyzed from the neck down is paralyzed. While the degree of their affliction is different, both people are paralyzed. More important, both people are considered disabled to such a degree that they require special aids and coping skills. Yet, when it comes to blindness people have a tendency to consider the totally blind to be blind, but view the partially blind, or partially sighted, to be able to see well enough to not be disabled at all. Add to that the fact many blind people appear normal. Their eyes are not shrunken or disfigured in any way, which makes it even easier for sighted people to wonder how the person involved can be blind. We like to ***see*** what is wrong with people. Not because we have some morbid sense of pleasure from seeing disabilities; but, because seeing the disability helps us to accept the limitations of the disabled person. In other words, when you see a person in a wheelchair, you can accept quite readily he has a disability. You may not even know what the problem is; but, you know there must be a problem or the person would not be in a wheelchair. Take a visually impaired person who does not yet use a cane or a guide dog, you can have a hard time understanding just how limiting their visual impairment is. The fact that many legally blind people refuse to accept their own limitations does not help this situation at all. They also refuse to use aids that would help them and their sighted friends or relatives, because, they are afraid they will ***look*** blind.

Yet, like the paralyzed people I used as an example, a partial or legally blind person is blind. Without getting too technical, I think it would help the reader a great deal to know what the different levels of vision loss are. This is a simplistic explanation. However, it will more than suffice in helping sighted people understand enough about blindness to realize that a person can be blind, and still ***see***. It is what a partially blind person does not see that can be dangerous.

A letter I received from Mr. Stan W. Gowin is representative of hundreds of others that I got during my research on this subject. Mr. Gowin wrote, "One aspect of blindness that is hard for the sighted community to grasp is the idea of varying degrees of vision loss. Most fully sighted people think that you can see or you cannot. As there are many who can see, but to a lesser or greater extent, from light perception, or no light perception, or to read with magnification, the ability to navigate well in restricted ranges of ambient light, etc., it might be helpful at least to mention these ranges of ***vision*** in your book."

Experts often refer to the first level of vision loss as ***visual impairment.*** The 1990 report from the Bureau of the

Census, U.S. Department of Commerce, stated that more than 20,000,000 people over age forty are afflicted with some form of visual impairment. The government expects this number to double in the next forty years. As the senior population grows, the number of people with age related visual impairment and blindness will also grow. Alarmingly, large numbers of infants who are born with AIDS, or who are addicted to crack cocaine have multiple disabilities that often include impaired vision.

A visually impaired person who has trouble seeing objects, may have trouble reading, and may see things hazy and blurry. A visually impaired person probably cannot have their vision corrected with glasses, and will use magnifying glasses or reading devices to be able to read. Sometimes just switching to large print will take care of their reading problem. When I went through the visual impairment stage, I used to have sighted friends who told me they saw worse than I did, but they seemed to manage just fine. What they did not take into consideration was the fact that their vision was correctable with prescription glasses, and my condition was not. Depending on the degree of the visual impairment, a person might even continue driving a car, or walking without any assistance.

As I pointed out earlier, it is what the visually impaired person ***does not see*** that can be dangerous. For example, a visually impaired person comes to a flight of stairs. They see the rail, they see what appears to be a staircase, but they cannot see the individual stairs. Nevertheless, because they ***think*** they are seeing everything, including the individual stairs, they step out and miss a stair. As a result, they take a tumble and fracture an arm. This happens to visually impaired people all the time. You cannot ***always*** tell by watching a visually impaired person walk down the street that they cannot see clearly. You might, for example, see someone you know who is visually impaired walk down a street without any apparent difficulty at all. They may find the store they want, due to the large print on the sign, and get in the front door without any difficulty. Once inside, this person may need the help of a sales person to find some product because they cannot see well enough to read the product boxes. This is one reason friends and relatives often think loved ones are lying about their visual loss. It is difficult for fully sighted people, particularly those whose minor visual problems can be corrected by wearing contacts or glasses, to understand how someone can see, but not see.

One young lady who wrote me, named Michelle, explained the problem she was having in this regard. "I tried to tell my friends what I am going through. Most of my friends told me that I did not seem to be any different to them since becoming visually impaired. I can still walk around, I can read most signs, and I go to movies. When I shop for new clothes, I pick out the colors I want. I can still match my own outfits by really focusing on the colors. Well, my friends still could not figure out how my life was any different from theirs, and, how I could, therefore, be visually impaired for real. Finally, I sat two of my closest friends down and asked them to tell me what they do in an average day. The first thing one of my girlfriend's said was that when the alarm clock went off, she turned it off and got up. That was all I needed to hear, and explained to these friends that I could not even find my alarm clock." Michelle went on to say that after a long talk with her friends some of them finally realized that she was not faking her visual problems.

Experts often refer to the second level of vision loss as ***low vision.*** The only difference between having low vision and being visually impaired is that a persons central acuity is affected, along with the entire visual field. I did not include any statistics or numbers on how many people may be afflicted with low vision in this level because experts usually include these numbers in the visual impairment category.

Low vision is usually more severe than mere visual impairment. It is usually the low vision level where many of the electronic assistive devices come into use. In fact, it is becoming more common to see people with extremely low vision using white canes and other mobility aids, and this really confuses a lot of sighted people. A low vision person will do something one minute which makes them identifiable as a person with severe vision problems. The next minute they will do something that shows they can still see to some degree. A sighted person would be very confused about why a person, who can readily see some things, would need a cane or other mobility aid to travel. Again, it is what the low vision person does not see that can be dangerous. An excellent example of this is a letter I got from a blind fellow named Tom. Prior too becoming totally blind, he went through the low vision stage. One day he was walking along a strip shopping center sidewalk, and without realizing it, he wound up in the back area where the shipping docks were. Because he had lost all depth perception, he was certain he was walking on a solid sidewalk. He could see the concrete. He could see the stores. What he failed to see was that he was walking off an eight-foot shipping dock. Another time he mistook a flight of stairs for a wheelchair ramp. Not seeing the steps, he walked off one into thin air and went cartwheeling down the flight of steps. While he reported no injuries, I think it is logical to assume he got some bruises and pains for his accidents. Again, because he was low vision at that stage, he could see some objects. It was what he could not see that got him into a dangerous situation. What is more important, he did not realize he did not see these things properly. Not perceiving the danger one is in makes the danger even more dangerous.

A letter I got from a man named Don Higgins on the Internet expresses the difficulties faced by those with low vision. He wrote, "Low vision is a very serious issue for many, many people. The biggest daily issues for me are the glare, tunnel vision, and adjustment to changes in light intensity. I have to wear very thick glasses with correction for removal of my natural lenses due to early cataracts at age thirty-nine, and prisms too correct for alignment problems following multiple detached retina operations. These glasses currently allow me to drive in the middle of the day if it is not raining. Early daylight, or late sunset, or bad weather, causes so much glare that I can no longer see well enough to drive. The glare in restaurants, due to the lighting is always a problem; and I try to get a seat with my back to the window so I can see people's faces and expressions during conversations. My tunnel vision is the real issue when it comes to walking to lunch, or anywhere in a crowd. I cannot see who is immediately next to me without turning my head to look directly at them. So, I like to follow people rather than walk beside them. Then, there are the low hanging branches I do not see at all until I hit them since my field of vision is about 40% gone above the horizon. Finally, there is the darkness that takes me thirty minutes to adjust to. Even then, I do not have good night vision at all. If I go into a dark restaurant, or into a dark hallway by myself, I often have to just stand there for a long time until I can see well enough to proceed, or until someone helps guide me. I always get to movies early, while the lights are still turned up. I go with someone who is fully sighted, or I do not go at all. ***Since I can drive some, and read well with proper lighting, other people often assume that I have perfect eyesight and cannot understand why I need a ride before sunrise, or at or after sunset to go somewhere.***" As one can see from Mr. Higgins letter, people who have visual impairments often have a great deal of frustration and difficultly with sighted people who do not understand their level of blindness or visual impairment. In fact, his condition is an excellent illustration of just how differently vision problems can manifest themselves. Mr. Higgins primary problem is tunnel vision. This is a condition that often allows its sufferer to see 20/20 directly ahead as if they are looking through a keyhole, but be partially or totally blind on all sides. It is something akin to a fully sighted person looking through a paper tube the size of a quarter. You can probably see straight out in front, but nothing to the sides, or above, or below that central spot without turning your head to see in that direction. That means that a person with tunnel vision, looking straight ahead, might be missing up to 80% of everything a sighted person would see without having to turn their head.

Another factor to consider in both visual impairment and low vision categories is this. The partially blind, or partially sighted, require individualized attention just like the legally blind, or the totally blind. Training people with visual impairment or low vision can often be a lot more expensive and complicated, according to the National Association for the Visually Handicapped. In fact, in a book written by Robert Scott, THE MAKING OF BLIND MEN, published by the Russell Stage Foundation more than twenty-five years ago, Mr. Scott stated the enormous waste of human potential by not making full use of all residual vision. He felt that, although visually impaired and low vision people far outnumbered the legally and totally blind, they were a forgotten group then. The National Association for the Visually Handicapped believes this fact is still true today. According to the N.A.V.H., the result is government programs for the visually impaired and low vision groups are extremely limited.

Experts often refer to the third level of vision loss as ***legal blindness.*** The latest statistics from the National Society to Prevent Blindness state that more than 900,000 Americans are considered legally blind.

Now, there is a specific explanation for legal blindness that goes something like this. "When the corrected visual acuity of the better eye is 20/200 or less, or one tenth of normal vision, or the visual field is 20 degrees or less, a person is classified as legally blind." It is at this level of vision loss a person can be certified by a doctor as blind by legal definition, therefore the term "legal blindness." At this level, a person can no longer drive a car, travel without some type of mobility assistance, or work at a career without some type of special training. Because there are so many different types of blindness, it is difficult to characterize how all legally blind people see. Many legally blind people can see shapes, colors, buildings, buses and other things. The problem is legally blind people have lost enough vision so that they cannot see a lot of the things they need to for safe travel, or to work, or to do things for themselves without having some way to cope. The vision loss is so great at the stage of legal blindness that even the most stubborn person usually realizes the time has come to use mobility aids. It is also easier to get government benefits like Social Security, job training, income tax credits, and the like. Not to belabor the point, but, it is something that needs to be said repeatedly. It is what a legally blind person does not see that makes coping skills essential for personal safety and daily living.

Experts often refer to the fourth level of vision loss as ***total blindness.*** A report of the National Advisory Eye Council of the U.S. Department of Health and Human Services suggests that there are roughly 100,000 totally blind people in America.

Many blind people were born totally blind. Others became totally blind due to injury, illness, or age. I don't mean to take anything away from people who are totally blind. I would not make the statement I am about to, except that, I heard it from so many totally blind people that I think it bears repeating. Understanding total blindness is easy for sighted people. For the most part, totally blind people do not see anything. So, sighted people find it much easier to deal with the totally blind than with blind people who can probably see something. I have had many totally blind people tell me they would rather be totally blind than partially blind. In fact, while taking blind rehabilitation at the Southeastern Blind Rehab Center in Birmingham, Alabama in 1995, I had a totally blind man tell me going totally blind was the best thing that ever happened to him. Don't misunderstand; he did not mean he would rather be blind than sighted. What he meant was, being partially blind was very confusing to him. He found it a blessing finally to be totally blind. Now he knew he could not see and coped with it. When he still had some vision left, he often made mistakes about what he could and could not see. His brain was receiving faulty information causing him a lot of problems.

There are other degrees of blindness I have not delved into here. You will often hear blind people say they have ***light perception***. This is a stage between legal blindness and total blindness. As the term implies, a blind person at this stage can tell day from night, unless it is a cloudy day. They can tell when lights are on in the house, if they are bright enough. Some blind people with light perception report that they can see very brilliant colors or shapes. Again, due to the contrast between light and dark, they can distinguish some shapes and objects.

I think most legally blind people are grateful for the vision they have left. I would rather see shapes, shadows, blurry colors, and sunshine than nothing at all. I can empathize with the man who had been legally blind and then gone totally blind. I have had to live with the problem of trying to determine what I can still see, and what I cannot.

The point is, 96% of all blind people have some vision. In many cases it can be difficult, and even dangerous, to trust what vision you do have, if you fall into any of the categories I have described in this chapter. Just because you still have some vision left does not mean it can be trusted, or that you are not blind or visually impaired.

For example, I was about to cross a street one day before I had a guide dog or a cane. I was doing what some of the low vision and legally blind people I have already cited were doing, that is, making the mistake of trying to cope with what sight I had because I did not want to be considered blind. I was in severe self denial because my family was not acknowledging my blindness. Of course, I felt I could slow the progress of my blindness by refusing to ***be blind.*** Well, I was blind. I nearly got run over that day because when I looked both ways I did not ***see*** any cars coming. Because I was depending on my remaining, faulty eyesight, I did not depend on my other senses nearly as much as I should have been. Because I could not ***see*** any cars coming, I started to cross and stepped right out in front of an oncoming pickup truck. The driver missed me only because he hit his brakes and swerved sharply to miss me. I was not only shaken to the bone, but, I sat there for more than a few minutes trying to figure out how I could look both ways with what vision I had left and still not see the oncoming traffic. That was the day I realized, if I were going to survive without being seriously injured or killed, I better start learning how to cope with what I could not see, and not just focus on what I could see. Being positive is one thing, letting a positive attitude blind one to reality, no pun intended, is dangerous and unproductive.

The best way for a sighted person to know what a blind person can see, or not see, is to ask them. In fact, blind people need to ask each other what their level of vision is. This may sound like simplistic advice. However, you would be amazed at how few sighted people ask a blind person just what they can and cannot see. This information can be critical to safety and well-being if you intend to be out with a blind friend or relative. Do not assume that, because a blind person you know can see a little, they can see everything they need to see. You would be surprised at how much your ability to do things can be affected by a little loss of vision. If you can see, but wear prescription glasses, you may know what I am talking about. Misplace your glasses and you probably cannot drive your car safely, or see to read a prescription medicine bottle, or walk to the store. Put your glasses back on and suddenly you can do all these things safely again. The problem for the legally blind is they cannot simply put on a pair of prescription glasses and see all clearly again.

This chapter should help explain why some blind people can see. It sounds like a contradiction in terms. When you realize that all disabilities, not just blindness, come in varying degrees of severity, it only makes sense that many blind people can see a little. What you need to find out as the friend or relative of a blind person is how much, if anything, they can see. Even more important, you need to find out, if they can see, what they do see well enough for it to be of any help to them. All the blind people I know would be happy to spend a few minutes explaining their degree of blindness to an interested person. While most blind people do not like to focus on the negative, it is critical for legally blind people to know what they cannot see and deal with it instead of just walking around trying to make the best of what they can still see.

If you would like to know what it is like to be visually impaired, low vision, partially blind, or totally blind, there are a number of ways you can experience blindness safely. As part of a classroom exercise, a teacher might have their students spend an hour "partially sighted." An adult might want to try this at home, or the office for an hour. Should you try this exercise please make safety your first concern. Do not injure yourself trying to travel outside unattended. If you do this exercise outside, let someone guide you so that you do not injure yourself. With those safety precautions in mind, you might want to experience blindness in the following ways.

Take a pair of swimming goggles and smear some Vaseline, Crisco, or other greasy substance on the goggle lenses. You can vary how much blindness you will experience by the amount of the substance you put on the goggle lens. Now, wear the goggles for an hour while you watch television, do your school work, or listen to your teacher. Try to see the blackboard, the television set, or try to take a walk holding someone's arm. Try to eat your dinner wearing your goggles. You will see what it is like barely to see a dinner plate, but not the food you are eating. If you want to be totally blind for a little while, wear a blindfold that does not let you look out from under it. (Be sure your goggles fit snugly, too).

This simple exercise may sound childish or ridiculous. Sighted people who work with blind people often go through similar training and know what it is like to be blind themselves. It is an excellent way for any sighted child or adult to see what it is like to be blind, and will also help anyone understand how you can still see something and be blind.

WHAT IS IT LIKE TO BE BLIND?

This is a very common question adults ask as often as children do. In fact, many of the letters I received dealt with this question. How does it feel to be blind?

Blindness generates a lot of feelings. One feeling all blind people feel is frustration. It is extremely frustrating to need to go somewhere, but you cannot go because the bus does not go the way you need to. Or, taxi fare is just too costly, and your friends are all too busy to take you. It is frustrating when you go out to eat and you cannot see the food on your plate or go to a movie and cannot see the picture. Imagine that you become a grandparent but cannot see your new grandbaby. Imagine becoming a parent and not being able to see your own beautiful new baby. You would be very frustrated, and rightly so. These examples are everyday occurrences for many blind people. I remember one young mother I went to guide dog school with. She was so frustrated she broke down crying during one or two days of the training. She was already six months' pregnant. As part of her guide dog training she was being taught how to manage using a baby stroller. Something all sighted mothers take for granted. There was no way this mother to be could push a baby stroller in the normal manner. It would stick out further than her cane, or her guide dog. In other words, the baby would arrive at any danger before the mother would know of the danger. So, the staff at the school was training her to ***pull the baby stroller behind her with the handle reversed so that the baby faced her back.*** Not only did she find having to pull a baby stroller from behind to be awkward and difficult, but, it put her precious cargo behind her. Her mother's instincts were to have her baby out front, just like any other mother does, for the protection of her baby. She was finally able to muster up the energy and resolve to learn how to manage the baby stroller that way. I don't think she ever got over the enormous frustration of having to handle her baby that way. I know she earned my admiration for coping with this difficult life situation.

Another extremely frustrating aspect to blindness really hits those men and women who are classified as ***partially*** blind, or partials. No one wants to be totally blind. Partially sighted, or partially blind people, are all happy to have some sight left. Being partially sighted can be far more frustrating than being totally blind. As I have stated in another chapter, a lot of totally blind people, with whom I have talked, agree with that statement. The frustration stems from the fact that partially blind people constantly have to rely on faulty sensory information from their eyes for everything they do. Continually receiving inaccurate information every second of the day can produce an incredible amount of stress and confusion for the partially blind person. For safety reasons, it is critical that the partially blind person filter every bit of information they receive visually to separate the inaccurate information from the accurate information before making each decision. Or, the partially blind person has to choose to use aids designed for blind people to supplement their remaining vision. Another part of the frustration stems from the fact that partially blind people frequently do not know they have received inaccurate information until it is too late, which can make being partially blind very dangerous. Again, totally blind people rely on feeling, hearing, and other senses to get their sensory information. They do not have to worry about receiving false or inaccurate information from faulty eyes. A totally blind person ***knows*** they cannot depend on their sight because they don't have any sight at all. Ignoring the faulty vision you have left to rely on your other senses is very difficult.

Blindness also makes a person feel lonely. I cannot tell you how often I have been out in public with friends or family and have everyone I encounter totally ignore me. I got many letters from blind people on this point. The problem is sighted people often assume, if you cannot see them, they cannot talk to you. So, instead of asking you what you think, or what you want, they will ask the person you are with. It is as if you are not even there. Nothing is more frustrating than being ignored when the person should be talking directly to the blind person concerned.

A letter I got from Fred and Patty Adams illustrates this point. Mrs. Adams wrote, "What my husband would like sighted people to know is that he wants to be addressed by them, instead of them addressing the sighted person standing next to him. Sighted people have a tendency to ignore him, or refer to him in the third person like he was deaf or incapable of making his own decisions or unable to answer their questions."

Another reason being blind can lead to loneliness is how

loved ones, friends, and co-workers relate to you. Unless you are a very outgoing blind person, it is easy to get shoved to the sidelines whenever something is going on. For example, one Christmas morning I was waiting to go to my father's house to join my parents and siblings for our annual Christmas get-together. I called my father and told him I was ready to go and asked if he would come pick me up. Since there was no bus service I could use, and I could not afford a taxi for the long distance involved, I needed someone to come pick me up. Well, my stepmother had other ideas. She decided, if I were not independent enough to get myself to their house for Christmas, then I just would not get to be there. Her ultimatum was show up either on my own, or not be there at all. I cannot describe the loneliness that engulfed my spirit that day as my entire family gathered for Christmas Dinner, opening presents, and having a wonderful holiday while I sat alone in my apartment trying to figure out what I had done to deserve such treatment.

While this is a personal experience, I can tell you such things happen to blind people every day. In my case, I had the problem of a family feeling I was not blind enough to need their help. A problem shared by thousands of other blind people.

Being blind can also make one feel inadequate. Most blind people do a fantastic job of coping with everything, myself included. For example, take the young mother I described in the last paragraph. She simply felt inadequate due to her blindness. What we have a hard time coping with, though, is how other people feel about us. In many cases, one's family and friends will totally ignore the fact you are blind. They insist on treating you as if you are sighted. When you cannot be sighted, or deal with people and situations like a sighted person can, you can begin to feel very inadequate. Unfortunately, ignoring a friend or relative's blindness does not make them sighted. In my own case, I do not have one relative on my side of the family that has ever acknowledged the fact that I am blind. In fact, as I point out in a later chapter of this book, in the course of my going blind, not one single brother, sister, parent, not even my adult son, ever acknowledged what I was going through. It was almost as if ignoring the problem meant that there was no problem. Unfortunately, I am still blind, and the love and support they might have given me to help through some of the more difficult times, when I was going blind or learning how to cope with blindness, was never there. It made me feel terribly inadequate. It was as if the fault lay with me, as if I was somehow inadequate; and, if I could only be more adequate, everyone would love me and all the problems stemming from my blindness would vanish. However, anyone who knows me will tell you that I am very adequate. There is really not much more that I could do to be any more adequate than I already am. While there are blind people who really are inadequate, due to lack of training or motivation, there are many such sighted people as well. There is no doubt that being blind can make you feel very inadequate, even if you are not.

Blindness has many positive aspects too. I cannot and do not judge people by the way they look. Unless a blind person has physical contact with you, or you describe yourself accurately, we don't know whether a person is fat or thin, tall or short, ugly or attractive, white or black. While we can tell a lot from the sound of footsteps and voices, smells and attitudes, for the most part, how you look or dress really does not have a lot to do with what we think of you. They often call this one of the blessings of blindness. Don't get me wrong; if I prefer dating thin women, I am going to find out if the woman I am dating is thin or not. You will find blind people are not nearly as prone to physical or racial stereotypes as sighted people are. You will not find blind people gawking at other disabled people. I cannot tell if someone I encounter is a burn victim with horrible scars all over their face, or if they are crippled and misshapen with palsy. I do know a blind person who was horribly burned. His disfigurement is no problem for me because I cannot see it. I hear his voice, I know his personality, but his physical appearance has no bearing on how I relate to him. Wouldn't it be nice if sighted people could relate to other people this way whatever their looks, disabilities, or skin color? Blind people do not get caught up in how other people are dressed. You might be wearing the most expensive suit made. You might be clad in diamonds from head to toe, but, if you do not tell me how you are dressed I would never know. You could just as easily be dressed in sackcloth. Most blind people are going to go by your voice, your personality, by whom you really are. In fact, we have a nudist colony near where I live in Orlando, Florida. I have never been there even though they have an annual open house for the public to come and see what a nudist colony is like. I frequently joke with friends that if I did go, I would be going by the people's voices and personalities, not by their appearance. I am not sure a sighted person could say the same thing about being in a nudist colony, whether for a visit or to live there. I do have a hard time imagining myself strolling nakedly with my guide dog through the nudist colony though. Since I use my feet to feel curbs and stairs going barefoot might be more hazardous than going without the rest of my clothes.

Do blind people dream? Yes they do. Speaking for those of us who used to be sighted, I can tell you despite the fact I am now blind, I dream in color. I see perfectly in my dreams. Since all visual images are recorded in the mind, the mind can play them back exactly as they were seen years ago, in dreams, though you may have since gone blind. I have had totally blind people tell me they dream. After I got my first guide dog, I found it interesting in my dreams I would still be with my guide dog, Frankie, running free in my dreams, just like any other sighted pet owner would be with their dog. As time has passed, my dreams have become somewhat mixed. Sometimes I am blind in them, and sometimes I am not. Even when I dream that I am blind, I am watching everything that happens. Since I was sighted at one time, I do have a lot of memories to draw on. There is no doubt my mind can continue drawing on these memories to construct dreams for the rest of my life.

A question I hear my totally blind friends get asked from time to time is how it feels to be trapped in total darkness all the time. Well, ironically, my totally blind friends respond they are not in darkness all the time. They point out that darkness is the absence of light, which is true. Since these particular friends have never been able to see, they do not know the difference between light and dark. They do not consider themselves in any kind of darkness. In fact, people who are totally blind now, but could see at one time do know the difference between light and dark. They report that they often see light, colors and images, and that they spend very little time in darkness. Think about it. Your brain stores information. When you see something, your eyes only transmit the information you see to the brain. The eyes do not turn the information you see into pictures or images. The brain is responsible for doing that. Since the brain lets you see the information, your eyes have only passed on the images that the brain stores. Even if you have gone totally blind and can no longer receive information through the eyes, the brain can call up what you have seen, and let you see it again. One young man who was totally blind started seeing, in his mind, brilliant flashes of white light. The flashes were so brilliant, in fact, that it scared the young man so badly, he had to get counseling to better understand what was happening to him. He, like many sighted people, was under the impression, if you went totally blind, you would never see anything again. He thought these brilliant white flashes meant he was going crazy or having a nervous breakdown. I have found I see brilliant flashes of green and red, blue and yellow. Since I was once sighted, I know what these colors are, and can tell you they are absolutely the most beautiful colors any sighted person could ever see. They rival anything I ever saw when I was sighted. Totally blind people also see what are called phantom images. While I was at the Southeastern Blind Rehab Center in Birmingham, Alabama, I underwent a psychiatric evaluation just like all the other blinded veterans who went there. The young woman who gave me the evaluation, Ms. Martin, asked me if I ever saw images. I asked her what kind of images did she want to know about. She said that she wanted to know if I ever saw people, or animals, or anything else walk by that I should not be able to see due to my blindness. My first concern was she was asking me a trick question. I mean, would YOU want to admit to a psychiatrist you thought you were seeing things? I said no, but, the truth was I did see things from time to time. It fascinated me when she explained to me that totally blind people see these images. That it is the brain recalling stored information and replaying it in the mind. As one can imagine, a lot of blind people who see these images think that they are hallucinating or having a nervous or mental breakdown. Ms. Martin's only interest in asking this question, I found out later, was to help those seeing phantom images understand it was a perfectly normal occurrence. So, not only do totally blind people not perceive themselves to be in total darkness as a sighted person would imagine, the vast majority of blind people report experiencing colors, lights and images.

One question I get all the time from children is, "Can I drive?" I explain that I cannot drive, although I used to drive, and enjoyed driving very much. In fact, it is one of the things I miss the most about being sighted. However, as my wife can tell you, I am an excellent backseat driver. I can tell from the feel of a car pretty much how fast it is going and if it is being driven properly. Fast starts and stops, sudden jerks right or left, tell me someone is driving a little on the wild side.

Blind people, despite popular misconceptions, do enjoy television and movies at the theater. Just because we cannot see the action clearly, if at all, does not mean we do not enjoy listening to the movie or television show. I am as big a Star Trek fan now as I was when I was fully sighted. I still enjoy television, movies, theater, concerts, amusement parks and all the other things I enjoyed when I could see clearly. I must admit I do miss ***seeing*** the action. I would like to know what the babes on Baywatch look like without having to trust my wife to tell me. She insists they are all ugly and have big noses. Blind people do not stop enjoying everything because they lose their sight. A lot of blind people do watch what they call ***descriptive videos.*** These are movies that are exactly what you would buy or rent at any video store. The portions where there is no speaking are described so a blind person can hear a description of what a sighted person would be seeing at that point. Keep in mind well into the middle of the Thirties families used to sit around the family radio and spend hours listening to radio programs which were actual weekly series. The fact there was not any picture to go with the story did not keep the sighted people in a family from gathering in the living room at night to ***hear a radio program*** complete with action, dialogue, and the like. So, it is not so far fetched that blind people would enjoy sitting in front of a television and listen to television shows or movies.

Another unique aspect to being blind is you find out there is very little you cannot do as a blind person, with the proper rehabilitation training. I owe a deep debt of gratitude to the men and women of the Southeastern Blind Rehabilitation Center in Birmingham, Alabama for helping me to realize this. They made such an impact on my life; I look forward to returning one day to get more training and rehab. It is my sincerest conviction that this facility is the crown jewel in the Veteran's Administration system of blind rehabilitation. Again, it is due to the wonderful and dedicated staff that works there.

I used to be an avid woodworker when I could see.

When I became legally blind, I was not too keen on putting my fingers and hands near a power saw blade to cut wood. I was also a hiker and backpacker. I loved walking every day. Because I could no longer see to take my walks, I had even stopped doing that. I had just had too many close calls crossing streets and falling into open manhole covers and the like to continue taking chances. So, I did what a lot of blind people do. I withdrew into my home and listened to television, radio, and talking books. I would only go out when my wife could act as a sighted guide for me.

When I got to the Blind Rehab Center in Birmingham, all that changed. Thanks to Robert Dailey I found out I could still do woodworking in Manual Skills Training. In fact, with his guidance, I turned out a wooden picture frame that rivals what any other experienced wood worker could do with full sight. When I went to the Blind Rehab Center, I wanted to find out if there was any chance that I could ever resume my hobby of woodworking. After making the picture frame, I know, with the proper tools, I can make anything I want to. All I need is the space for my workshop.

Thanks to the dedication and caring of Harvey Clark in the Orientation and Mobility section, I found that, with proper cane use, I could still take all the walks I wanted. While I now use a guide dog, I keep my cane skills sharp in the event I need my cane again. I will never forget any of the people at the Blind Rehab Center. I will especially remember Harvey Clark. He was a professional in every sense of the word and treated me with the utmost respect and dignity. He listened to what I had to say about my goals and desires. In fact, I still chuckle when I think about my first day or two with Harvey. I had gone to the Blind Rehab Center with one specific goal in my mind, to stop running into door posts, walls, and stumbling on stairs. I am a large framed man. When I run into anything, there is always a considerable impact; and, I was tired of sore shoulders and elbows. Harvey went right to work on these problems. I always looked forward to every training session with Harvey. I hope, when I do return to the Blind Rehab Center in Birmingham, Harvey is still working there.

I don't know whether to thank Gerta or not. She improved my house keeping and cooking skills. She taught me how to sew and do dishes without vision. Whatever chances I had of convincing my wife I could no longer cook, clean, or make the bed vanished after Gerta got hold of me. I had this mischievous notion that I could go home and tell my wife I was not supposed to do any more housework. When I jokingly mentioned this plan to Gerta, she let me know she would be calling my wife to tell her she had trained me in every aspect of cooking, cleaning, laundry, etc. Gerta did make that phone call to my wife. All joking aside, Gerta saw to it I can live totally independent should I ever need to do so. Instead of being a burden to my wife, I can work hard around the house, even if I do not want too sometimes. Thanks to Gerta, my wife frequently comes home to find her dinner already prepared, or the laundry done, or the house vacuumed. No doubt about it, Gerta is probably the most popular person with sighted wives.

I also owe a deep debt of gratitude to everyone else at the Blind Rehab Center. They all helped me learn what it is like to be blind, and how to cope just like any sighted person does. They also taught me to do many other things that seem to shock people for one reason or another. I backpack with my guide dog and wife. Some of the areas we backpack in have alligators and rattle snakes. I mean we really get out in the wild areas. I don't know what my guide dog will do when we encounter an alligator, a black bear, or a rattlesnake; but, I think we will handle any such encounter well. Again, it is because the men and women at the Blind Rehab Center have given me the confidence I need to go out and do those things again.

I am involved in bodybuilding. I may not be a contender right now, but, I can do one intense weight workout under the supervision of a personal trainer. Except for being blind, I am in exceptional health. Yet, I meet people who are amazed that a blind person, me in this case, is in a gym lifting weights. Why? Except for being blind I am just like any other sighted bodybuilder as far as being able to lift weights is concerned. I do have to cope with a few problems like how much weight I am lifting. Since I cannot read the weight on the plates or the machines, someone helps me with that. Ironically, very few blind people go to the gym or fitness center to workout because they believe their blindness somehow prevents them from doing so. The blind people who do go to the gym or fitness center and pursue better health and fitness are proof blind people can do just about anything they want to.

If you are the sighted spouse of a blind person, or the sighted parent of a blind child, never forget that blind people are a lot more capable than sighted people sometimes think they are. When I do meet a blind person who can hardly do anything for themselves, I usually find that the problem stems from the way this person was raised, not any lack of inherent ability on their part. In other words, many blind people are raised to think they cannot do a lot of things, so they don't. I am reminded of one person who attended a blind rehab center at the age of forty-five. On arriving at the Center, he began to rely on nurses, staff members, and other blind people to do simple things for him like pouring him a soft drink. Can you imagine being in your mid-forties and not knowing how to pour yourself a soft drink? It is incomprehensible to me as a blind person. I can imagine how it looked to the sighted people who encountered this unfortunate man. His only problem was no one had ever showed him how to cope with his blindness. Everyone in his family had always waited on him hand and foot ***his entire life.*** Unfortunately, he had decided there would always be someone there to wait on him and take care of his every need. I shudder to think what is going to happen to this man when his family is no longer able to wait on him in this manner. He will be in a managed home of some kind with other disabled people who were never taught how to take care of themselves.

As this example shows, it is critical for blind adults, and blind children, to realize their full potential. There is just absolutely no reason that an otherwise healthy blind person cannot do anything they please, within reason. A blind child cannot grow up to be a race car driver, or an Air Force jet pilot. Yet there are blind lawyers, doctors, bodybuilders, business administrators, teachers, writers. You name it; blind people are doing it. It is time blind people realize there are a lot fewer limitations on them than the sighted world, or other blind people, would have them believe. As I have already stated, blindness is a state of mind, as much as it is a physical disability. While blind people cannot control the extent of their blindness, we can all control our state of mind.

THE DARK SIDE OF BEING BLIND!

There is a dark side to being blind which needs to be dealt with. I feel it is important for sighted people to know about the negative aspects of what it is like to be blind. Again, it is not the purpose of this book to be a forum for whining. Understanding the negative aspects of what it is like to be blind will help the sighted reader as they relate to blind people in the workplace, at church, or as friends. So, I have given the information in this chapter in the spirit of helping sighted people realize there are some areas where they can help make the life of a blind person easier.

Relatives often make life the hardest for a blind person. They either tend to make us out to be totally helpless, or go to the other extreme and refuse to acknowledge we are blind. This attitude leaves many blind people without any help or consideration at all. There is a middle ground. I hope this chapter helps sighted people have a better understanding of what that middle ground is.

An excellent example of this is some of my own relatives. While I do not want to offend, I know many of my blind friends have had the same experience. If talking about my experience here in this book helps other sighted families deal with their blind loved ones better, then talking about my own experiences will have been worth it.

There is nothing to describe what it is like to go blind, or be blind, and have that fact be ignored by your loved ones. In the last seven years, as I progressed from severe visual impairment to legal blindness, I have not had one single family member on my side of the family offer one word of comfort. Not one has asked a question to help them understand my blindness, or made any attempt to see if there was anything they could do to help me cope with the situation. When my left eye had to be surgically removed in 1993, I did not get one single card or flower from anyone on my side of the family. Not one person from my side of the family, who was close enough, bothered to visit during my recovery. When I spent a month at the Blind Rehab Center in Birmingham, Alabama in 1995, I never got a single phone call or card from anyone on my side of the family. When I came home with my first guide dog, not one single relative told me how happy they were for me. A brother who lived near by never even bothered coming over to meet my new guide dog. One might argue, of course, that I must have done something to alienate my relatives. That any blind person with this problem has had to have done something to alienate their loved ones. I am sure this is true sometimes. I got literally hundreds of letters about this problem from other blind people. I cannot believe that every one of those other blind people are all guilty of alienating their relatives. I think that in most of these cases the families think by refusing to acknowledge a family member is blind, then that family member is somehow ***not*** blind.

I would also respond that when a loved one is going blind, has just become blind, or is blind, it is time to show a little love and caring no matter what kind of relationship there has been before the blindness. When a blind person's family ignores their blindness, victories in rehabilitation, their pain and suffering at losing a very precious sense, sight, it leaves a deep and abiding pain that just will not go away. It makes the blind person feel they don't exist and are simply not worth anything. After all, if my blindness is not important enough, or serious enough, to warrant the love and caring of my family, then, what does that say about me? It says I am not important enough, or going through enough, to warrant the love and caring of my family. I don't care how well grounded you are mentally or emotionally, having your blindness totally ignored by your family is devastating. There is no excuse for this type of behavior by any sighted family member or members.

This is a form of denial many sighted family's experience concerning a blind loved one. If they deny the blindness, then their loved one is just not blind anymore. That attitude is terribly wrong, of course. The result of this denial is it is deeply hurtful to the family member who is blind, or who is going blind. No one who is blind should expect their family, relatives, or friends, to smother them with sympathy or attention. However, to totally ignore some loved one's blindness is often devastating emotionally, and always puzzling. If you have a blind loved one, and you have been ignoring or denying his or her blindness, now is the time to let him or her know you know. Give them encouragement, give them love. Most of all, ask how they are doing once in awhile. This gives your blind loved one a chance to tell you what coping skills are used with their visual loss. It gives loved ones a chance to know they are not alone in coping with blindness. It will also give your blind loved ones the courage to cope, with all the problems and frustrations blindness brings, for another day. Don't let past squabbles or differences stand between you. Blindness is a devastating condition. It deprives a person of a great many things that were an important part of life. Any person who is going blind, or who is blind, needs every bit of love and support they can get. There are more practical aspects to this problem. I got a letter from one blind man who was absolutely devastated because his son was not speaking to him. In fact, his son would not write him, call him, visit him, or even respond to his requests for prayer. In the course of this dispute between this father and his son, the man went from being legally blind too only having light perception. The last chance he had to see his son, with any kind of clarity at all, slowly went away as his vision decreased. Where his son could have spent some time with him and let his father enjoy what he still could see of him, his son ignored him; and, this father lost any chance he had of ever seeing his son again. What had the father so devastated is this was an opportunity lost forever. Even if he gets back on speaking terms with his son in the future, he cannot *see* him again.

In another letter, a woman described a similar situation with her younger brother. They had apparently never been close, or spent much time together. Both were busy working and taking care of their respective households. Then, something happened in the family that drove a wedge between the two. The younger brother would no longer have any contact at all with his older sibling. As the older sister's vision went from legally blind to totally blind she longed for the opportunity to spend time with her brother. She wanted to see him, or what she could see of him despite her legal blindness. She wanted to etch the memory of her brother's face into her mind so that when she did go totally blind the memory would never fade of how her brother last looked. According to this woman's letter, she went totally blind without ever being able to see her brother again. There is no way that the pain this lady feels will ever be erased. Again, even if she and her brother have a reunion, she forever lost the one last chance she had to see how her brother looked.

Let me give you a similar example of what I am talking about. After years of denying the way my own family had treated me concerning my blindness, I finally sat down one day and wrote my stepmother a pointed letter. (My real mother died in 1981, and my stepmother had been my mother since I was twelve years old). In the letter, I politely and lovingly told her I did not understand why she had never shown one ounce of concern or sympathy for my blindness. I asked her why she had never written to me, or called me, to tell me she did care about my blindness, and she was praying for me and hoped only the best for me in coping with my blindness. I made it a special point to write the letter so it required a response so there was no way my mother could not answer. Well, I never got an answer. My mother totally ignored my letter. It was as if I had never written or sent it, as if my mother did not know I was blind. That is about as total a denial as one can get from a loved one concerning their blindness, or any condition. Yes, I know she got the letter.

I got many letters in my research from blind people who had parents who had openly voiced their embarrassment at having a blind child. That a parent could say something like that to a blind child, even though these were grown blind children, is shocking. There are parents out there who are embarrassed they have blind children, just as my relatives may be embarrassed they have a blind relative. I cannot tell you how devastated the people who wrote me these letters were. They were blind; there was nothing they could do to change their blindness; and the one thing they desperately needed was the total love and commitment of their parents and relatives. If you as a sighted parent ***ever have the urge to tell your blind child they embarrass you, please don't.*** Blindness is tough enough to deal with when you have parents and relatives who are totally loving and supportive. It is miserable when your blindness embarrasses your parents or relatives. Remember, anyone can go blind at any age. If you went blind, you would not want anyone telling you that your blindness embarrasses them. Blind people have a hard time, as it is, not being self conscious about their blindness. I do clumsy things occasionally like knock over a glass of tea in a restaurant, or drop food on the floor, or wear a shirt wrong side out. All blind people have had these things happen at one time or another. We do enough to embarrass ourselves and know that some of the things we do must sometimes embarrass the people we are with, but, never voice that embarrassment if you feel it. Try to put yourself in the blind person's shoes. It is not easy being blind. The most important fact is that a lot of sighted people get clumsy and do some of the same things blind people do.

What is it like to be blind? It is everything I have dealt within this chapter and more. The most important thing to remember about what it is like to be blind is this. Blind people are people. I got hundreds of letters asking me to get this point across to sighted people. We are real people, talk to us, not around us. Tell us when you are standing there so that we can say hello without speaking to thin air, or being rude by passing you. Remember, we are blind; tell us what we need to know instead of waving or gesturing with your hands.

If you are our waiter or waitress at the restaurant we patronize, tell us where our drink and plate is. Tell us when you take something away or put something new at our place. Friends and family, tell us when you walk away so we will not stand there talking to ourselves for ten minutes. Blind people are people. While that may seem obvious on the surface, it must not be. Every day, blind people are ignored, dealt with as if they are sighted, and shunned by friends and family who don't know how to deal with a blind friend or loved one. We have to deal with sighted people who just don't want to take the time to talk to us and find out more about how our blindness affects us.

To end this chapter, I want to make a statement I have heard many other blind people make. It may sound startling too many sighted people. I am just as happy as a blind person as I was as a sighted person. Blindness is a state of mind. Don't get me wrong, if you are blind, you definitely are physically blind. Blindness is a devastating disability; but, attitude is everything. I meet paralyzed men and women who are miserable with life, and everyone around them. I also meet paralyzed people who are an inspiration to be around. I meet people who have no arms or legs who are bitter with the world, and angry with God. I also meet people who have no arms or legs who accomplish their goals with just as much success and enthusiasm as a physically complete person does.

So, what it is like being blind depends a great deal on the blind person. Sighted people will meet bitter blind people who hate God for letting them be blind. They will also meet blind people who accept their blindness and live their lives to the fullest.

No one wants to be blind. I have never talked to a blind person who does; but, we are blind and can deal with it. The eyes are only one part of the whole body, albeit a very important part. Even without ones eyesight, a person can still feel, hear, walk, talk, and do nearly every thing a sighted person can do. The important thing to remember is, as a sighted person, there is a lot you can do to make being blind a lot easier on anyone you know who is blind. There are a lot of things you can do, as the loved one of a blind person, to make their lives more fulfilling and emotionally stable. Blindness is a lot like life; it is whatever you make of it. Those of us who are blind can always use a little help from our friends, no matter how independent and adjusted we are.

BLIND PEOPLE ARE BLIND!

This is the topic I got the most mail about. It sounds like a contradiction in terms to say that blind people wish sighted people knew they were blind, it really is not. Almost every day, a blind person encounters sighted people who do not take their blindness into account. While blind people want to be accepted as normal in every other way, there are some things we blind people cannot do. In these areas, we need the help and consideration of our sighted friends.

A good example of how sighted people forget we blind people are blind is how sighted people frequently greet the blind. I was walking with my mobility instructor at the V.A. Blind Rehab Center in Birmingham, Alabama one day. He was walking far enough behind me that it appeared as if I were walking by myself. After crossing a street intersection, he came up beside me to tell me how a driver had waved frantically for me to cross the street. When I did not cross the street, the driver had apparently gotten angry with me and started making some rude gestures with his fingers toward me. Of course, I was oblivious to the entire incident because I could not see his gestures. The point is I did not see his gestures because I was blind. That fact should have been evident because I had my white cane with me. During my mobility training at the Blind Rehab Center, this experience was repeated over and over again.

I have had the same experience when I am out walking with my guide dog, Frankie. Almost everyone knows a guide dog when they see one. Just this morning, while we were out walking, we had such an experience. We were waiting for the proper traffic pattern to cross over from one side of an intersection to another. I knew there were some cars at the intersection; but, it was just not the right time for us to cross. And we were not crossing. Finally, I heard a woman yell at me, "Hey, don't you see me waving for you to cross. Can't you see that there are cars waiting for you to cross?" In fact, I had not seen her waving. Like so many sighted people, this lady found it is easy to forget that blind people cannot see you gesturing at them.

It is also very common for people to walk up to blind people and stick their hand out to shake hands without ever telling the blind person they have their hand out. Then they get offended when the blind person does not extend their hand to complete the handshake. I have gotten so used to this phenomenon that I can usually sense when someone has their hand out and so I extend mine. Sometimes, I find out I was mistaken, and then I feel foolish. It just works better all around if sighted people would remember to tell blind people when they extend their hand to greet them.

Another good example of this problem is when I go out to church, or to a meeting. A member will try to hand me something. Instead of saying, "Here, Harry, I have something for you," the person will just stand there holding it out waiting for me to take it. Or they say hello to me without telling me who they are.

Don't misunderstand what I am saying here. I know, and most other blind people know, that this is totally unintentional on the part of sighted people. I have had many sighted people tell me later that they simply forgot I could not see, and that they felt a little foolish. I guess this problem is positive in that it shows many blind people cope so well their sighted friends sometimes forget that they are blind. It can still be an annoying problem, because we blind people do not want our friends thinking we are rude or stuck up by not waving back, or responding to their gestures.

So, if you know a blind person, or encounter a blind person out in public; remember, blind people cannot see. It is important to *tell* a blind person what you want them to know, or to tell a blind person your hand is extended in greeting, or when you say "this way" also include which way "this way" is. Is it left or right? Or, is it up or down? A blind person has no way of knowing which way "this or that way" is unless you tell them.

Another really common situation is where I give my guide dog the command to find a door for me at the mall or a store. People are nearly always courteous enough to open a door for us; but, they don't tell us they are holding the door open for us. Not knowing someone is holding the door open, I reach out and feel to see if it is open or closed. I then inadvertently wind up touching the person where I should not, and wouldn't if I knew that they were there. It is just a matter of sighted people forgetting blind people cannot see them standing there. It would help the blind person if people would announce they are there and holding the door open.

I, and a lot of other blind people, often find that our waiters or waitresses will come to our tables and take items away, or add items without telling us where they put them. This can cause some frustration if a blind person is trying to find something that was there a minute ago, but has since been taken away or moved. The appropriate thing to do would be to tell the blind patron when anything is added or removed from their table. In fact, when a waiter or waitress does remember I am blind, and helps me in this way, I always add a little to their tip. That is how much I appreciate this courtesy. Ironically, in the last year, I have had only one waitress take the few seconds to tell me where my food and drink were so I would not have to figure it out on my own. I think her extra courtesy was not only a compliment to her, but to the restaurant where she worked, GREEN STREETS in St. Augustine, Florida.

Even blind people, who still have some residual vision, need to have specific directions such as left, right, up or down. They need to have people tell them when they are handing them something, or offering them a handshake. Remembering blind people cannot see may sound like a contradiction in terms. However, it is an easy thing to forget, and is one of the most common problems blind people deal with. We hope this book will help remind all our sighted friends we cannot see.

HOW DO BLIND PEOPLE GET AROUND?

There are a lot of myths and misconceptions about how blind people get around. When I went blind, I thought everyone knew that blind people used white canes, guide dogs, and other mobility aids to travel. I soon discovered I was wrong.

I was trained to use a white cane at the V.A. Blind Rehab Center in Birmingham, Alabama by a fantastic mobility instructor named Harvey Clark. He was professional in the extreme, and he was sensitive to my needs as a newly blind person. During his course of training, I had an opportunity to travel with fellow blind students on weekend walks around town who were also learning to use a white cane. I learned two important lessons very quickly.

The first lesson was that most of the sighted community did not know much about how blind people travel with a white cane. The second lesson I learned was that a lot of

blind people do not know very much about how to travel with a white cane. This second fact contributes a lot to the myths and misconceptions sighted people have about how blind people get around.

Traditional canes used by blind people are white nearly their entire length. The last five or so inches are painted red to let any observer know a blind person is using this cane. The blind person using it may be legally blind, or totally blind. By properly using the cane, a blind person can find his or her way just about anywhere they need to go. The emphasis needs to be on the word *properly.* If a white cane is not used properly, the blind person can put themselves in danger. Improper use of a white cane can really confuse any sighted person watching. To make matters even worse, there are blind people who have the attitude that since the cane gets them where they are going who cares how they use it. Well, there is a right way, and a wrong way to use a white cane. The right way of using a white cane helps blind people travel safely, or as safely as is possible in a fast-moving society. The wrong use of a white cane can get a blind person killed.

To clear up any misconceptions a sighted reader might have about proper use of a white cane, here is a short lesson. The top end, or the handle, of the cane should be held at the waist by the blind person. They should grip the handle firmly, but not too firmly, in case the tip hits a rock or a crack in the sidewalk. If it does, it will ram into the user's stomach and that can hurt. Held with the right grip and angle of the wrist the cane will break loose just enough from the grip to slide harmlessly up the front of the chest of the user. Yet the user never loses their grip enough to drop the cane. Although, eventually, I think just about every white cane user has dropped their cane. The cane has a wrist strap, but it is highly inadvisable to use this wrist strap when out walking. The reason for this is that if the cane gets hit by a car and a blind person is wearing the wrist strap, their arm goes flying along with the cane's momentum causing the arm to be seriously injured or broken. If the cane gets stuck in a train door, a car door, or elevator door, a blind person can be dragged along with their cane and seriously injured or killed. Without the wrist strap around the wrist, the blind person can easily let go of the cane to ensure their own safety.

They point the cane down to the walking surface at the proper angle. The blind person moves the cane back and forth from one shoulder to the other to check for any obstacles in their immediate walking area. The idea is for the cane to check the area where the blind person will next step. If used properly, the cane will find, and let the blind person know, of any cracks, holes, poles, curbs or anything else that might cause a problem for the blind walker. When the cane does encounter something, it is up to the blind person to decide what to do next? A cane can only find an obstacle, and only then at ground level. It cannot tell its user what to do about the obstacle. A traditional white cane does not detect overhead obstacles; although, there are laser canes that shoot out a laser beam to locate and signal the user about overhead obstacles. Due to their high cost, laser canes have never come into wide use.

Now, one of the problems blind people have using the cane in public is sighted people often ignore the cane. I have had people walk right up on my cane, knock it out of my hand, and just keep right on going like nothing happened. I have also had sighted people grab my cane while I am going up or down stairs or curbs thinking they will help guide the tip of it for me. What this does is takes away all the sensitivity in the cane leaving the blind person with no way to feel what the cane feels anymore. **You should never touch a blind persons cane unless you ask them first, and get permission to do so.** Should you inadvertently grab some blind persons cane they will most likely ask you to let go immediately, and you should. A blind person may even be sharp or blunt in their request for you to let go of their cane. Do not be offended if they are blunt or sharp. A blind persons cane is an extension of their person, and it is critical to their safety. No matter how sharp or blunt a blind person might be with you, if you grab their cane, they should always use courtesy in any reprimand.

When you see a blind person with a white cane at an intersection, you might be tempted to offer assistance. If you are tempted to offer assistance, there is a right way, and a wrong way to do so. The wrong way is to walk up and grab a blind person, or their cane. Never walk up and grab a blind person or their cane. For all they know, you could be a purse snatcher, a rapist, or a mugger. When I was in Smithtown, New York attending guide dog school to train one of the female students related a story to me that really brings this point home.

She was standing at an intersection waiting to cross. While listening to the traffic patterns, something all blind people do to determine when they should cross, two men walked up to her and grabbed her arms. She immediately went into a fighting frenzy and was furiously beating the men with her cane, her purse, her fists, and all the energy she could muster. In just a split second she had one man down on the ground, pounding his head with her fist. The other man tried frantically to explain to her they were police officers. Well, she had no way to know what they were, since she was blind and could not see them. Based on the way they just walked up and grabbed her, she decided she ought to keep right on pounding the one she was sitting on. It apparently took some convincing and struggling to get her calmed down and convinced they were really police officers. As it turned out, they thought she needed help crossing the intersection and had decided to give her the help she needed. They now know that the proper and polite thing to do is to approach the blind person and then ask if they need assistance without grabbing anything. They also learned it is the safest thing to do.

Now, I hope this true story has not scared any sighted readers away from offering assistance to a blind person who might really need help. Again, there is a right way, and a wrong way to find out if a blind person needs help or not. The right way to offer assistance is to walk up to the blind person and announce yourself, then, ask them if they need assistance. If they do, they will tell you. Then, ask how you can assist them properly, and they will tell you exactly what they need you to do. This technique allows you to help where they need your help. Do not be offended if the blind person declines your offer of help. It just means they know where they are going and what they are doing, even if it is not readily apparent to a sighted observer. Never let the fact that one blind person declined your help keep you from offering your help to other blind people. There are blind people who do need help from a sighted passerby. You just have to remember not to walk up and grab a blind person and start dragging them off somewhere.

To help sighted people understand why a blind person might remain standing at a curb or an intersection longer than a sighted person would, here is a quick lesson in how blind people cross streets and intersections. (The ones who know what they are doing). When a blind person gets to an intersection, they have to rely on what their cane is telling them about the curb location and where a crossing might be. They have to rely on their hearing to tell them ***when*** crossing it is safe, and how much time they have to cross. Sighted people can look at the crossing sign, or the traffic signals, or the traffic itself to determine when they can cross. A blind person cannot rely on any of these visual cues.

Now, imagine you are blind. You have arrived at a busy intersection and want to cross to the other side. The first thing you have to find out is what ***kind*** of intersection it is. Is it a four-way stop sign? Are there traffic lights? How many traffic lights are there? Is there a left turn signal in any of the lanes, at any of the lights that might allow cars to cross right in front of where you need to go when the light turns? If you are on the other corner, are there any right turn signals that would allow cars to cross into your path if you step out too soon? Can you begin to get the picture of what a blind person has to figure out before they can decide when to cross an intersection? That is just the beginning. Once the blind person has all of this information, they have to decide where their ***parallel*** traffic is. This is the traffic they are going to want to cross with. When I am standing on a corner with the intention of crossing in the same direction the traffic is going, the traffic moving my way on my immediate left is my ***parallel surge.*** If there is no right turn lane, I need to wait for this surge, and then go when I know that my parallel surge is moving.

This is the reason sighted people will observe a blind person stand through several traffic cycles without making any attempt to cross. The blind person has to listen to enough traffic cycles to determine where their proper surge is, when it goes, and when they can safely cross. Even then, a car will run a light, or make an improper turn nearly hitting a blind person while they are crossing, even though, the blind person is crossing at the proper time.

Again, it is better to ask a blind person with a cane if they need assistance than to leave a blind person who does need help standing at a corner for a long time. There are a lot of blind people who do need assistance. Just don't be offended or surprised if they politely decline your offer.

A word to sighted drivers; if you see a blind person standing on a street corner waiting to cross, don't try to wave or honk them on. They cannot see you waving, and they have no way of knowing whether you are honking at them or the car in front of you. If a blind person does not go when you think they should, there is probably a very good reason that they are not going. If you see a blind person crossing and you realize that you have inadvertently blocked off the crosswalk, don't panic. Stay where you are. The blind person will tap your car with their cane and go around you. Depending on how they have been trained, they might feel their way around the front of your car, or go around the back. Having a blind person feel of your car with their hand or their cane will not hurt your car or your paint job. After all, you are the one blocking the right of way. Moving your car forwards, or backwards, might just cause an accident. Just think about how you would feel if you had to cross a busy intersection with your eyes closed, and nothing but your hearing and a white cane to tell you what was going on; and, you found someone was blocking your right of way. Since a blind person has no other way to tell who is in their way, or how to get around the car, they are going to have to touch it with their cane and hand to determine what to do.

Another tip for sighted people to use when they see a

blind person with a cane is the cane is going to touch everything in its path. That is how a white cane works. If you insist on standing in front of an oncoming blind person using a cane, you are going to get touched by the tip of the cane. Let the blind person know you are there ahead of time if you do not want to be touched by the tip of the cane. It will not hurt you. Some sighted people act offended when a blind person touches them with a cane, despite the fact they stood there without saying a word to let the blind person know they were there. It is very common for sighted people to remain quiet when we approach them. I don't think this is always intentional on the part of the sighted person. It may just be that the sighted person does not know what to say, but, say something. It really helps a blind person know what is going on around them. By letting a blind person know you are there, you prevent inappropriate touching. For example, when using a guide dog, it is common for a blind person to check for the sides of the door entry with their right hand to make sure they are going to clear it, and to praise their guide dog for stopping at it. If you are standing in that door way, and to my right, you are going to get touched by my hand if you do not say something to let me know you are there. How short or tall you are will determine where I touch you. You would not believe the sighted men and women who will just stand there and watch as you reach out to feel the door entry, and never say a word to let you know they are there. Then, after you touch them, they make a big fuss about the fact that you inappropriately touched them. Listen, I know there are a lot of jokes out there about blind people touching everything in their paths for the fun of it. The truth is most blind people hate to touch people just as much as people hate to be touched. The rule is if you ***can*** see, and I ***cannot*** see, it is your responsibility to tell me you are there. If you don't tell me you are there, then, it is your fault you got touched.

Unfortunately, there are a lot of blind people who do not use their white canes properly. They cross intersections at the wrong times afraid they will appear stupid if they wait out a few traffic cycles. Some blind people use white canes that are way too long and wind up tripping other people. Other blind people swing their canes in such a wide arch that they would need a two-lane highway to travel down. If you, as a sighted person, encounter a blind person, who seems to be using their cane wrong, give them the benefit of the doubt. We can hope someone will tactfully encourage them to get the training, which is readily available, to use their cane properly.

Here is an interesting fact. Blind children do not, for the most part, use white canes. The theory is that a blind child should be escorted by a sighted adult at all times, making the use of a cane unnecessary. Although, as of this writing, there is some experimentation going on to teach blind children how to use a cane. It is my hope in the future that blind children using canes will become common place. Although, it will be even more essential to teach proper cane technique so they do not form bad cane use habits in childhood, making these habits harder to correct later in life.

There will still be the need to be with an adult until they reach an appropriate age. There are, however, many blind children who, at the age of ten to thirteen, would be ready to use a cane alone if they had been trained to do so.

The other way blind people get around is by using a guide dog. A guide dog is a highly trained animal whose life is dedicated to working with a specific blind person. We usually call a guide dog and a blind person a "guide dog team." Teamwork is the key word; because, it takes the skills of both the blind person and the guide dog to travel safely.

This brings us to another common misconception about the blind and how they travel. Most people think the guide dog does everything; but, it is not true. For example, if the team needs to cross an intersection, it is the blind person, not the guide dog, who decides when it is time to make the crossing. The blind person would use the same techniques with a guide dog that he or she would use with a white cane, determine the type of intersection, and proper traffic surge to cross on, and decide when to make the crossing.

The advantage of using a guide dog is if the blind person makes a mistake and tries to cross at the wrong time, the guide dog knows to ***willfully disobey.*** In other words, the guide dog will not cross, and the blind person knows something is wrong, to try again when it is safe. A white cane has no way of willfully disobeying its user; and, so, a blind person without proper training can easily make a mistake in crossing. This is why drivers' should always keep an eye on a blind person crossing in or near their lane of travel. Blind people are killed all the time because they made a mistake crossing an intersection, or, because of driver error.

Another advantage to a guide dog is when it comes to something called a ***traffic check.*** This is when a vehicle comes screaming around a corner or through an intersection oblivious to any pedestrians crossing. Believe it or not, some of these drivers hit and kill blind people out of sheer carelessness every year. The fact that it is a blind person with a cane does not slow such drivers one bit. A guide dog is trained to come to a dead halt when such a driver comes through, hopefully preventing its blind user from being hit and killed. This again, is something a white cane cannot do.

A guide dog can, and does, alert its blind user to curbs, overhanging tree limbs, outcropping bushes, light poles, and protruding cars. If a child leaves a tricycle on the sidewalk, the guide dog will stop and give its user an opportunity to feel for it, and then move around it. So, if there is a guide dog team in your community, you will see the team stop frequently for obstacles. You will also see the blind person feel to find out what the obstacle is. He or she will then direct their dog to get them around the obstacle. If the blind person does not know, or cannot figure out a way around the obstacle, the guide dog will find a way. If the obstacles are on the guide dog's side, the dog will usually go ahead and make its way around them, if doing so does not push their user into any other obstacles.

There are several other important facts all sighted people should know about guide dog teams. You should never pet any guide dog without asking the blind person first. Since it is best that other people do not pet a guide dog, the blind person will probably say no, although, occasionally a blind person will let you pat their guide dog ***only on the shoulder.*** Never pet a guide dog on the head. That is where their master pets them for doing a good job when they are done working. A guide dog is a dog, and this ***love reward***, petting on the head, will get them excited. If you try to sneak a pet in when you should not, you will distract the guide dog; and, the user may have to correct the dog to get it back in its working mode. If you pet a guide dog, and its user has to correct it, that is your fault. You should not get angry with the blind person. It is essential, even critical, that a guide dog keeps its mind on its work. Even when sitting or lying completely still, if a guide dog is in its leather harness, it is working.

Now, when a guide dog is at home and out of its working gear it is, essentially, off duty. In that situation, members of the immediate family, or very close family friends, may be allowed to play with the guide dog. In the case of my own guide dog, I do have several very close family friends that I do let play with my guide dog when he is at home, and out of his working gear. When I go to the gym for a workout, I make one exception. I let my personal trainer pet him on the shoulder for a moment and say hello to him. This helps my guide dog, Frankie, follow the personal trainer around the gym from one piece of equipment to the other more readily. On even rarer occasions, when I am out in public, I may let a small child pet my guide dog, again, only on the shoulder, if they are afraid of dogs. I make this exception because I want children to know a guide dog is not an animal they have to be afraid of. It also gives me a quick chance to tell them about guide dogs and what they do.

One of the biggest problems we guide dog users have when out in public are other peoples pets. Even in areas where they require that pets be on a leash, my guide dog and I frequently encounter dogs that are running loose in the community. The reason this is a difficult situation for me and Frankie is we never know which of these dogs will attack us, and which ones will not attack us. Since we have already been attacked once, it is something always on our minds. While we do not live in fear of another dog attack, until the dog shows his or her intentions, we do not know if we are going to get to pass unhurt or not. I have listened as loudly barking dogs charged out of their yards at us, as if they were going to attack, with people all around us saying nothing to stop the dog's charge or quiet its barking. If you know you have a guide dog user in your community, be aware of the danger of having an unrestrained dog barking at or disrupting a guide dog team, or, heaven forbid, attacking the team before you can put a stop to it. This is not just in the best interest of the guide dog team. It is your best interest as well. The dog that attacked Frankie and I was seriously injured, and the vet cost to the owner was around $2000. In addition, the owner was responsible enough to realize his dog was at fault, so he was out the $600 vet bill for Frankie. Not being a litigious person, and being grateful the owner took responsibility for my vet bill, I had no intention of suing the man. I would have been within my rights, however. Worse still, had his dog killed or maimed my guide dog, I would have been without a guide dog for months while waiting on a list for another one. Then, there would have been the enormous emotional blow that losing my guide dog would have been to me since Frankie is my friend.

Another point I think needs to be made here is that it is cruel to tease a guide dog, or a guide dog team. In my opinion, you have to really be a mental moron to do so. Yet, no community is so small that there is not someone in it who takes pleasure in taunting and teasing guide dogs and their blind users. These people are definitely in the minority, but, cause enough troubles in any given day to be extremely annoying. My own community offers an excellent example of what I am talking about.

I lived in a small apartment complex with about fifty units. Every day when my guide dog, Frankie, and I would go outside we would encounter dozens of friendly, courteous neighbors who treated both of us with dignity and respect, and who knew better than to tease a guide dog. We had two young men who lived in one of the other buildings who went out of their way to cause problems for me and Frankie. When I would take Frankie out to go to the restroom, or to break, these two young men would whistle at him, and do other things to distract him from his work. They generally succeeded in distracting him enough to cause me to correct him. Their antics did a thorough job of disrupting Frankie's breaking schedule.

The extraordinary thing about these two young men was they were not children. I had several neighbors tell me they were at least eighteen year's old. If they were not brave enough to come sit on their front stairs and distract my dog, they would sit inside their apartment window and do it from inside the safety of their room.

One, day I finally let their taunting get under my skin. I looked in the direction the whistling was coming from, and just point blank asked them if they were the ones who were whistling at my guide dog. When they did not answer, but only whistled more, I turned around and directed Frankie to take me to them and he headed their way. Of course, when we got to the stairs where they always sat to do their dirty work, they were gone. A neighbor later told me they had quietly gotten up and tip toed into their apartment with an enormous grin of delight on their faces at having caused me and my guide dog so much consternation.

The point is it does not take a very brave, or a very bright, young person to mock and taunt a blind person. I could not see them, and I could not catch them, even if I wanted to. One has to wonder how boring a life these two men, and others like them, must lead to have nothing better to do than sit outside and mock disabled people as they walk by.

The reason I think this is important enough to bring up over and over again in this book is this. Teasing or distracting a guide dog team can be very dangerous. I have had other young people about the same age as these two young men try to call Frankie across busy highways while they stood on the other side. Frankie is too well trained to take their bait. If they distract him, he could easily miss an oncoming car; or, I could be injured falling, or, getting hit by some overhanging objects.

I have a word of advice for these young people, and others like them. Grow up for a minute and walk over and meet the guide dog team. I would be happy to introduce these people to Frankie and tell them how he works. They might discover a small measure of respect and admiration for Frankie, his intelligence, and his dedication to me. Then, instead of wasting their time taunting blind people and guide dogs, these people could be out meeting young women or get involved in sports.

There is also a new device that helps blind people get around which can be used with a white cane or a guide dog. It is called "Strider." This is a device developed for the military which pinpoints the location of a person to within twenty feet. That may not sound very accurate. Still, if I am walking two or three miles, and I get lost or disoriented, knowing my location within twenty feet would be a real lifesaver. That is exactly what this device will do. Carried in a backpack the user can type in their location on a laptop computer that talks. The unit then relays the information to an orbiting satellite. That satellite then processes the information and relays it back to the blind person's computer. The computer will then verbally tell the blind user where he is and will even tell him how to get where he is going. Like many such devices for the blind, this unit costs at least $4000. Which, unfortunately, puts it out of the reach of many potential blind users.

While this chapter has not gone into every detail of how blind people get around I hope that it has helped the sighted public understand that blind people can and do get around very successfully. In fact, I have an interesting point to make about just how well blind people do get around. I live in Orlando, Florida just northeast of many major theme parks like Disney World, Sea World, and Universal Studios. Every year a number of tourists are killed being hit by cars because they are walking too near the highway, or crossing at the wrong time. Yet, it has been many years since a car has killed a blind person in my area. The reason is sighted people are not careful enough. Sighted people assume they can cross when they really cannot, or, that a driver will see them in time to miss hitting them. Blind people who are trained properly in travel skill's make no such assumptions. As a result, far fewer blind people are killed in such accidents than sighted people. In other words, blind people are often safer travelers than are sighted people. When a blind person is injured by a driver, it is often the driver's fault, rather than the blind persons.

For example, Frankie and I were walking through a park near our apartment one day. The road we were walking on was a rural road. That is, it did not have any sidewalks so Frankie and I were walking along the left edge of the road facing the traffic. This is the technique used by guide dog teams walking on a rural road. The road was straight and without any obstacles. This meant any driver approaching us would be able to see us for about one hundred yards in advance. Since we had walked this route hundreds of times before I was not too concerned about being hit. Most cars passed us with plenty of clearance. Today we would not be so lucky.

I heard a vehicle approaching about every one minute due to traffic in the park that day. Suddenly, and without any warning, a van hit me on the right side of my body. This was the side facing the traffic. I was knocked violently to the right with Frankie's harness anchoring my left arm in place. I can still remember feeling the side view mirror and mirror brace on the van bending a little from the force of the impact. My body protected Frankie from any of the impact. His weight kept him from being pulled up or injured.

Luckily for me, the van was only going about ten miles an hour. Still, I was left stunned and aching from the van hitting me. The whole right side of my body was in intense pain. Nevertheless, I did not black out or fall down. I did hear the van stop about fifty feet from where the driver had hit me. After a few moments hesitation the van drove off. I could not believe the driver was unaware he had just hit a pedestrian. Still, the driver left the scene which meant I was on my own insofar as any injuries.

I took a moment to size up my injuries and realized I had been hurt. Still, I felt I could limp my way back to my apartment and get my wife to take me to the Emergency Room at the local hospital. As I was attempting to limp back home a car pulled up beside me and a man told me he had chased down the driver of the van and called 911. I wound up going to the hospital to get evaluated. Surprisingly, the Highway Patrol did not even issue the driver of the van a ticket. He claimed he never saw me, and never heard a thud when he sideswiped me.

To make a long story short, this accident ended my bodybuilding and aerobic activities. I spent the next eight months in excruciating pain from an injured shoulder, back and right leg. I had to fight the man's insurance just to get my medical bills paid. Amazingly, incidents like this are all to common for blind people.

The most common problem for blind people walking are drivers who pass to closely. If you are driving through a parking lot or down a rural road and see a blind person with a cane or a guide dog, leave at least four to five feet between them and your car. If you cannot leave that much room, then stop until they have passed you. I have had many cars come so close to me as they passed, their side view mirrors touched me. On occasions they touched me so hard as to sprain or injure my hand or wrist. Amazingly, not one has ever stopped to see if I was alright. I have also had dozens of cars nearly back out over me and my guide dog as we walked through apartment or store parking lots. I have also been hit and injured walking on sidewalks when bicycles try to pass me to closely. In one case the impact injured my left shoulder and left hand so badly I could barely use my guide dog for weeks.

In another case, a car came into our apartment parking lot and went speeding into a parking spot just in front of where I was walking. The car came within inches of hitting me and my guide dog. In another instance, a car backing out of an apartment parking spot actually backed into my guide dog. If I had not realized what was happening and quickly pulled my guide dog out of the way he would have been killed. I would have probably been run over too.

If such incidents were rare it would be bad enough. Unfortunately, such incidents are all to common for blind people. I have blind friends, who like me, have been run over four and five times. One blind lady I know was paralyzed and will spend the rest of her life in a wheelchair, in addition to being blind. All because a driver was in to big a hurry to avoid hitting and injuring a blind pedestrian. What every driver needs to understand is this. If I get seriously injured because of a driver's careless driving, I am going to sue that driver for everything I can get. In fact, I did sue the van driver who hit me because I had no intention of paying medical bills he caused me to incur. ***If nothing else motivates a driver to avoid hitting and injuring the blind it should be the fear they will lose everything they have in a law suit***. Believe me, being blind is tough enough without having to worry about being run over and killed every time a blind person takes a walk.

Just do any blind person you see or encounter the courtesy of letting them use their training to get around. If you find out that they need assistance, be sure to render that assistance in the manner described in this book. If you encounter a blind person when you are out driving, leave enough room between you and that blind person so as not to hit and injure them.

WHAT BLIND PEOPLE WISH OTHER BLIND PEOPLE KNEW ABOUT BLINDNESS!

One of the most surprising discoveries I made as I read the letters sent to me by blind people was how many of them wanted other blind people to know about blindness. That sounds like a contradiction in terms. After all, how could a blind person not know enough about blindness or other blind people? Yet, I have had many experiences with other blind people that confirm what some of these letters were talking about. A lot of blind people need to know about other blind people, and blindness.

I am reminded of an incident while I was at the V.A. Blind Rehab Center in Birmingham, Alabama. At the time, I was having a lot of trouble with the indoor glare from florescent lighting. This is a problem many legally blind people have. The glare from such lighting can interfere with what sight you do have left. This is one of the reasons you see so many blind people wearing sunglasses indoors and outdoors. By cutting the glare, many blind people can then continue to use what vision they have left to see shapes or outlines, or whatever it is they still can see.

I had one older man, who was also at the V.A. Center for rehab, come to me at least a dozen times and tell me I should not wear sunglasses indoors, that wearing them messed up my appearance. I was always polite and explained to him that running into a door or wall could also mess up my appearance. That the glare was such a problem for me I found it necessary to wear the sunglasses even indoors. I was only one of several people who had a problem with the glare and was not the only one wearing sunglasses inside.

This brings up the reason that some blind people feel that other blind people need to know more about blindness. There are many different forms of blindness, and many different causes. Different types of blindness require different remedies. So, one person's blindness may not cause a problem with a glare, indoors or outdoors, while another person's blindness does. Ironically, while a blind person may be very knowledgeable about their own form of blindness, they may not have any understanding of another person's type of blindness at all. This leads to one blind person trying to make all the other blind people they encounter into clones of themselves, thinking that what works for them ought to work for other blind people.

Another very good example of why blind people need to know more about blindness is an incident that also took place at the V.A. Blind Rehab Center in Birmingham, Alabama. They called our group into an assembly one afternoon to hear a short speech from the gentleman after whom they had named the hospital. After this totally blind war hero had concluded his remarks, we all stood to applaud. When the applause ended, I sat down thinking the man had been escorted out of the room. Instantly, I heard a fellow vet next to me chastise me severely for not continuing to stand for such a great man, who, it turned out, was still in the room. My fellow vet was legally blind, but could still see enough to tell the man had not left the room yet. He assumed that because he could see the man was still present that I could too. Again, he thought it was his job to make every other blind person conform to his level of blindness. He did not mind chastising anyone he thought was not measuring up to his own abilities or vision level.

This man also gave me another example of how blind people should be more tolerant of each other's levels of blindness. He and I went out walking one day to practice our cane skills with two or three other blind veterans. I was very good at continuing in a straight line because I checked myself against the edge of the sidewalk frequently. Because the cane was pointed straight out in front of me, it acted as an aid in traveling a straight line. As I was walking up a hill, I heard him yell at me from behind, "Harry, how is it that you can walk such a straight line if you can't see?" What a question, I thought. Here is a fellow blind person suggesting, just by the wording of his question, that any blind person who can walk a straight line with his or her cane, must be able to see to do so. Considering I had spent three weeks in serious training so I would know how to walk in a straight line with a cane, I was astounded to hear his question, especially since he had been getting the same training to do the same thing.

Another good example of the blind needing to show a little more understanding toward each other is a line of conversation currently going on online, with a guide dog list I subscribe to, on America On Line.

A partially blind man recently posted a lengthy letter on the guide dog list telling everyone how he felt guilty, when he went to guide dog school, because he still had some residual vision left. He felt, like many partially blind people do, if he got a guide dog some more deserving totally blind person would be deprived. I know; I also went through this stage. Feeling this way is extremely common for the partially blind.

Well, this man did get a favorable message back from me, and from another blind person on the list. We both told the man that he was more than deserving of a guide dog; and, he did not need to feel guilty because the guide dog schools usually dealt with prospective blind students on a first come, first serve basis.

His letter, and our responses, began an intense tirade of letters from a number of totally blind people who did not like "partials" at all. Partials, of course, being blind people with some residual vision left, and totally blind people being just that, totally blind. Several of these tirades absolutely astounded me. First, they showed an incredible lack of understanding on the part of the blind people who posted them about the different degrees of blindness and the problems faced by the partially blind. Second, the postings suggested that the totally blind people writing them were just too quick to assume things about the partially blind.

For example, one post was from a blind woman who was relating how she and a partially blind man were in her house one day visiting. The partially blind man's guide dog was, according to this totally blind woman, at least twenty feet away from its user. When the dog got up and moved around, the partially blind man corrected it. Well, that was all the proof this totally blind woman needed to prove this man had too much useable vision left to even need a guide dog, or to be classified as blind. In her words, he had to be able to clearly see his dog to know the dog had gotten up and moved. I guess it never occurred to her that this man could have listened to the rattle of his dog's tags. Which is the way I tell when my dog is moving. Or that this man might have even been able to see enough to see his dog as a "blob of blur." In which case, the man would have seen the dog well enough to know he moved, but, not well enough to distinguish the features of the dog. No, in her opinion, he could see so well he could not be blind.

Another letter posted to this guide dog list related an

experience a totally blind lady had while at guide dog school. She and the other students were on the school's bus headed for a training session in the downtown area. As the trip progressed, a partially blind student apparently made the announcement that she knew where they were because she had "timed" the trip so far, and according to this timing they would have arrived at a certain point. It was the opinion of the totally blind student that, since the partially blind student had not lived in this area, she could not possibly have known enough about the area to be timing how their trip was progressing. When another one of the totally blind students expressed some disappointment at not being able to do as good a job at timing their trip as the partially blind student, this lady informed that totally blind person there was no way the partially blind lady could be timing anything. She had to be reading the signs to see where they were, which meant she really was not all that blind. What was the basis for this totally blind lady's opinion that a partially blind student could not be timing their trip? It was the fact that she, a totally blind person, had lived there for years and did not even know how to time the trip. It was also the contention of this lady that there was nothing worse than partially blind people who had learned the terminology of the blind; because, this made them able to appear more blind than they really were. In other words, the lady saying she was timing the trip was using the language of the blind to fool everyone into thinking she was really blind, when in fact, she was reading signs to see where they were. Could it be this partially blind lady really did know how to time her trips? Since this is one of the techniques taught in blind rehab, I would suggest to the reader this partially blind lady was using the techniques taught to her at blind rehab, which should be obvious to a blind person of all people.

To go to blind rehab, or to go to guide dog school, a blind person, partial or total, has to submit medical documentation of their vision loss. It is not a matter of calling up the guide dog school and telling them you are blind and you want a guide dog. Medical documentation has to be provided ***proving*** your blindness. Of course, this lady had that covered too. I posted a message to her asking her how people with too much sight could get into a guide dog school. Her reply was that guide dog schools were so worried about discriminating against the visually impaired due to the American's With Disabilities Act that they were now taking everyone just to protect themselves. Checks with a number of guide dog schools on this matter verified this lady was not correct in her belief.

Why, then, is it partially blind people are allowed to have guide dogs at all? This is a question I have been asked by both the totally blind, and sighted people. It is a very fair question. Here is the answer.

At one time, only totally blind people were eligible for guide dogs, or blind rehab, or training with white canes. Then, someone realized if they extended these mobility aids and the training to use them to the partially blind they would have an easier time learning to adapt to them because they did have some residual vision left. While most partially blind people will never go totally blind, many do. It is apparently much easier to learn to use a guide dog ***as you go totally blind, instead of waiting until you are totally blind.*** Then we have the consideration that it is what the partially blind person ***does not*** see that is so dangerous to their safety. I hope that totally blind people will consider that whenever they feel the need to berate or condemn the partially blind.

My point is this. Totally blind people who resent partially blind people are, I hope, in the minority. It is arrogant in the extreme to assume, that, because you cannot time a trip in an area that you have lived in all your life, then no one else can either; or, that, because a blind person can tell their guide dog has gotten up and corrects them, they are not really blind. In both these cases, I think the totally blind people doing the complaining are making up for their own shortcomings concerning their own coping skills. By attacking other totally blind, and especially partially blind people, these blind people take our attention away from their own shortcomings, which makes them feel better.

Just as the partially blind man berated me at the V.A.Rehab Center for the Blind, these totally blind people were busy berating their partially blind brothers and sisters, something that is not necessary at all.

I did get a lot of letters from blind people that wanted other blind people to know things that are really more a matter of personal preference than the way it has to be. For example, I got many letters from blind people bemoaning the fact that people always wanted to buy them dinner. This offended them because they felt like a charity case if someone else bought their dinner. They felt all blind people should be taught to turn down people who offered to buy them dinner just as a matter of principle. While I agree that people should not buy blind people dinners simply because they are blind, I do enjoy being taken out to dinner occasionally at someone else's expense. I also return the favor at every opportunity. The best advice I can give here is, if you offer to buy a blind person dinner and they turn you down, don't push it. Let them buy their own dinner. Don't be afraid to ask the next blind person if you can buy their dinner. I think this is one of those topics that should be left to blind people as individuals. If I am offended at other people wanting to pay for my dinner it does not mean all other blind people are also offended.

I got a lot of letters pointing out that blind people ought to observe the same courtesies toward each other that we expect sighted people to abide by. For example, it is quite common for blind people to leave a room without telling their blind friends they have departed. As a result, we keep right on talking to them. Blind people are also bad about not telling an oncoming blind person that they are directly in their path of travel. When I was away at guide dog school, we had a woman, a fellow student, who would stand in the hall until one of us ran into her. I tend to be humming, singing, or musing to myself as I walk along. I knew she could always hear me coming long before I ran into her; yet, she would never warn me she was in the way; and, my extended hand would wind up in contact with various of her body parts. A little word of warning would have let me know she was standing there; and, I could have avoided her.

One of the most common gripes I got from blind people was how some blind people are prejudiced against each other. I heard from blind people who were shunned by other blind people because of their blindness. That sounds incredible, doesn't it? I have encountered this form of prejudice myself, which apparently stems from the fact these blind people resent the fact they are blind. To be blunt, they loathe themselves. So, they take this out on other blind people by avoiding and shunning them.

One has to wonder, with all the work that needs to be done for the blind and disabled, why the blind can be so insensitive to other blind people. If we cannot respect each other's individuality and choices for coping with our blindness, how can we expect the sighted world to do the same? We can't. No one blind person, or group of blind people, has the right to tell any other blind or disabled person how they should do what they do, or what mobility aids they should, or should not use. When we, the blind, attack the use of say, disabled parking spaces, all we do is give more ammunition to sighted businesses that want to find ways to eliminate disabled parking spaces from their businesses. They cannot at the present time. If groups made up of the blind, or militant blind individuals, keep demeaning the use of disabled parking spots, or guide dogs, just to cite two examples, anything is possible.

Another interesting situation in the blind community is the use of braille. In the sighted world, everyone has a choice of using standard print, or different levels of large print. In the world of braille, there is standard braille, micro braille, and large cell braille. The problem is there are almost no publications or materials available in large cell braille. This discourages many older blind people from ever learning braille because they cannot feel the dots of standard braille. When I learned braille, I could not find one course in large cell braille. I had to learn with standard dot braille. Yet, I could read large cell braille with ease. When I wanted to get a braille bible, there were no large cell braille bibles. The argument was a large cell braille bible would simply be too cumbersome. A standard dot braille bible requires about eighteen volumes; and, I estimate a large cell braille bible would require about fifty volumes.

When one realizes only about 10% of all blind people read braille, one wonders if it is not because they need large cell braille materials; and few are available. While writing this book, I polled every organization for the blind that provides braille materials and could only find one or two that had any materials at all in large cell braille. In the sighted world it would be unheard of to have so few materials available in large print for the sighted. Yet, organizations that cater to the needs of the blind, including organizations made up of the blind, have yet to seriously address the almost total lack of large cell braille materials for the blind. Talk about a positive project for an organization to undertake. Making large cell braille available on a wide scale to the blind and helping promote education in this more easy to read form of braille could easily revolutionize blind rehabilitation.

I received some letters pointing out the single most important issue is how blind people treat other blind people, although the connection may be hard to grasp at first. The point is how some blind people seem to loathe showing appreciation to the sighted community for things they do for the blind. What does this have to do with how the blind treat the blind? Well, if I let the sighted community do something for me as a blind person, then refuse to be grateful; or, go around berating the very people who helped me, I might just wind up hurting another blind persons chance to get that same help.

For example, I got into quite an argument one time with a gentleman about guide dogs. It was his contention that guide dog foundations are not charities. In his opinion, they are not charities, and the blind people, who get guide dogs from them, do not owe them any debt of gratitude. After all, if they are not charities, then they are money making enterprises, he argued. He was not given his guide dog by a charity who should be thanked. It was his contention he got his guide dog from a profit making machine, and the profit the school was making was the only thanks they deserved. To offer gratitude for being given a guide dog would be admitting to having accepted charity. That would, after all, make him a charity case. Well, the fact is all the guide dog schools I know of are charities. Guide dogs are provided at no cost to blind people. Sighted people and organizations usually sponsor them who sponsored them as an act of charity. Frankly, if I had to pay the $25,000 it cost to train and raise my guide dog, Frankie, I would not have a guide dog; because, I could not afford one. I am not going to play mind games with myself, or others, to try to make the gift of a guide dog anything other than what it was, a charitable gift. Blind people, who feel used by guide dog charities or the organizations sponsoring them, ought to use a white cane, or pay for the dog. They should be very careful their lack of gratitude does not influence some organization or per-son to donate their charitable dollar to another worthy charity, thus depriving some deserving blind person of a guide dog.

If I were to include every suggestion I got about what blind people wish other blind people knew about blindness, I would have a whole book on that one topic. We blind people really need to work on how we treat and deal with each other. Instead of trying to make every other blind person fit into our mold, we should have the same respect for them as we expect others to have for us. As I have said before, when blind people attack and malign each other just to push their own agenda, we cannot expect the sighted community to treat us with dignity and respect. We cannot ask of others what we are not willing to do for ourselves. It is high time individual blind people and organizations made up of blind people stop and think a minute before stating opinions or agendas that affect ALL blind people.

One last case in point, which illustrates what I am trying to say here, is this. I have had a number of blind people tell me that they have gone to some length to make it known in their communities they do not want, and do not need, disabled parking spots near businesses. Further, they refuse to get, and will not use, disabled parking signs because, they do not consider themselves mobility impaired. A particular organization that acts as an advocate for the blind also takes a position on disabled parking which states blind people should not use disabled parking areas. The reason being to do so admits to being disabled.

What a crock! If blind people are not mobility impaired, then I would like to know who is. Sure, with good cane skills or a guide dog, most blind people get around quite well, in fact, sometimes, better than sighted people. However, for those blind people who do not consider the blind to be mobility impaired I suggest the following exercise. Leave your cane, your guide dog, your sighted guide, and every other mobility aid you have at home and take a trip to the store. A blind person trying this exercise will discover they cannot do it. Why? Blind people are mobility impaired.

I cannot think of a more dangerous place to walk than through a shopping center parking lot, cars constantly passing, backing out and pulling in and not always watching where they are going, I might add. Being able to park in a disabled spot as near the entrance of a store is just as important for a blind person as it is for someone who is wheelchair bound. Now, if some blind people out there do not want to use disabled parking spots because they think it diminishes them as a blind person, that is their choice. To try to push that position for all other blind people is ludicrous at best, and dangerous at worst. It is just such issues that demonstrate the kind of infighting and pushing of special agendas that go on between different blind groups and people all the time. Then, we expect the sighted community to deal with us fairly, and with an open mind. We expect service providers to consider our needs and wants when they plan services and programs to meet our needs and interests. Yet, there are blind people out there who refuse to do the same for other blind people.

I keep this thought in mind at all times in dealing with my blind brothers and sisters. I am a unique individual, and so are each and every one of my blind colleagues. What works for me may not work for some of my blind friends. What works for them may not be what I need. So, I respect their right to do what they feel is best for them. I expect them to respect me for doing what I think is right for me.

There is an even larger issue at work here. Blind people are part of a larger, more global disabled community composed of the paralyzed, the deaf, and others. When we take issue with something like disabled parking spots in our community, we are not just affecting the blind. Our actions are affecting every other group of disabled people, too. How tragic it will be if ever some activist group of blind people succeeds in curtailing certain rights that were fought for long and hard by the entire disabled community. Do not be foolish enough to think that it cannot happen.

Again, if you, as a blind person, think it is demeaning to use a disabled parking spot, then park in a regular parking spot. If you, as a potential guide dog user, think it is demeaning to accept charity from a guide dog school, or a sponsor of a guide dog, then do not get a guide dog. If the blind membership of your particular organization thinks guide dogs are a cop out for being truly independent, then stick with a white cane; but, at least, respect the rights of other blind people to make use of disabled rights and mobility aids that make their lives a little easier.

If you are a totally blind person who thinks that partially blind people, or partials, should not be getting the same level of benefits, training, or aids that totally blind people get, remember it is what a partial does not see that can make life very dangerous for them. Even according to many totally blind people, partials may have a tougher time than the totally blind do. Sometimes being able to see something is not the blessing you think it is. Receiving faulty information every moment your eyes are open can be frustrating, dangerous, and extremely taxing on the mind.

DON'T BEGRUDGE BLIND PEOPLE THEIR RIGHTS!

Disabled people, including the blind, have won certain rights through hard fought battles. Yet, they are still denied many of the rights that the disabled, and the blind, have won. Worse, non disabled people often begrudge the blind and other disabled people for these rights. As I pointed out in the last chapter, sometimes blind people begrudge other blind and disabled people their rights.

The reason sighted people should not begrudge blind people, or any other disabled group, their hard won rights is simple. ***You never know when YOU might be blind or disabled and need the very rights you resent so much now.***

Take Christopher Reeves, the movie actor. Christopher always respected all the rights of the disabled. Who would have ever guessed Christopher Reeves, the hero of the Superman movies, would one day become a paraplegic? He helped the disabled as a fit, non disabled person, and now he deserves to use every right the disabled have. Many people resent these rights, like disabled parking spots, being exempt from pet deposits if they use a service animal for mobility or assistance, or getting financial assistance from Social Security. Unfortunately, many businesses do not respect the rights the disabled have won.

Let me give the reader a couple of examples. I talked to a young woman the other day who works out at a local gym. The gym has the obligatory disabled parking spot. It is located clear around to the back side of the gym. Such parking spots are supposed to be near the front door, or as close to the front door as it is feasible to have them. Repeated requests to this establishment to move their disabled parking spot to the front have been refused on the grounds that it discriminates against non disabled members who might want the convenience of parking near the front door. This reminded me of one evening I went to my own gym to a workout. When my guide dog and I got to the wheelchair ramp, which was the only access to the front door of the gym, we found one of those huge four wheel drive monster trucks parked right on the ramp. Not only did it block the way we needed to go, but, the man driving the truck had taken two parking spots to park. Instead of parking somewhere out in the parking lot, where he had more room, he had used the disabled parking spot, along with the regular parking spot next to it. Keep in mind, this man had come to the gym to a workout. Yet, he could not walk a few extra feet to park his truck where it would not be in some disabled persons way.

Another example is an experience one blind couple had in Texas. According to this couple, they had decided to move to a more upscale apartment community than the one in which they had been living. When they went on a tour of the apartment community they wanted to move into, they told them that they would require a $500 pet deposit, and $250 of the pet deposit they paid would be forfeited when they moved out. The husband explained to the manager that guide dogs were exempt from pet deposits because they were not pets, but service animals. He was then told by the manager that she ***had*** to charge them the pet deposit because not doing so would be reverse discrimination to sighted people who do have to pay a pet deposit. According to this couple, no amount of explaining would change her opinion she had to charge them this pet deposit. Being a little on the wily side, they decided they would make sure they had been accepted by this apartment community before pursuing the matter any further. They did not want the apartment management turning them down because they would not pay the pet deposit, when they might have been accepted otherwise. They wanted some time to get their facts and information together before presenting the matter to the management a second time. Meanwhile, they had to go ahead and reserve their apartment by signing a lease and paying all their deposits, including the $500 pet deposit.

When they finally did get their information together to present to the apartment management, they found out, not only was it unlawful for an apartment complex to charge a blind person a pet deposit for a guide dog or other service animal in their state, the law they had cited had been in effect since 1971. After the management consulted with the same State agency this couple had and were informed that they were breaking the law, they refunded the couples $500. The fact is they should have never charged the deposit in the first place. Although, in this case, the couple was convinced the business was not familiar with disabled rights, or access laws for service animals and guide dogs.

Here is another example of how many disabled rights are ignored by sighted people. I often get to a business, or back to my own apartment, only to find someone parked in the disabled spot who does not have a disabled parking permit. Since most disabled parking spots have additional room on the left and right of the vehicle, it is much easier for me and my guide dog to get in and out of the car when we are in a disabled parking space. Not only that, but, when we get in or out of the car, I need to either remove or put on my guide dog's harness. This requires him to stand while I bend over and buckle the harness under his chest. When my wife has to park in a regular parking spot, this can be an almost impossible task due to the lack of room between cars. I also frequently get out of our car in a disabled spot to find that some sighted person has parked their car right in the access space that leads up onto the sidewalk. Since they clearly mark these spaces with bright yellow paint and diagonal lines, anyone parking in such an access space knows exactly what they are doing. Since I can squeeze between cars, although with some difficulty at times, I can usually get around this problem; but, someone in a wheelchair is totally denied access when anyone parks in this marked access space next to the disabled parking space. I would like to think this lack of caring about the disabled is unintentional on the part of sighted people. However, the access spots are just too clearly marked to be mistaken for a regular parking spot.

No, anyone parking in such an access point simply does not care whether a wheelchair bound person, or other disabled person, can gain access to the building or walkway in question. I have had sighted people watch sighted, non disabled people, park in disabled parking spaces, or in these access areas, then glance back and forth as they walked off toward the door apparently making sure no one saw who they were.

The point is this, disabled people would prefer to not be disabled. When we experience non disabled people trying to prevent us from using our rights, it is a bitter reminder we are living in a society not quite as enlightened as we thought it was. I can guarantee you one thing. Any disabled person would gladly give up every disabled right they have if they could trade their disability for a normally functioning body. I would gladly trade my blindness for a sighted person's eyesight. If I were sighted and had a pet, I would happily pay the pet deposit, and would not harbor any hard feelings for the blind people with guide dogs, or disabled people with service animals who did not have to pay the pet deposit. In fact, when I was sighted, I did not harbor any resentment for any disabled group, or their rights. I was always glad to park somewhere else besides the disabled parking spot; nor, would I begrudge the disabled people who did have a parking spot near the door that right.

I have a permit for a disabled spot now that I am blind. It is a permit I use when my wife and I are out together. When I am not in the car, she does not use the disabled spot or the parking permit. It is only used when I am in the car with her to meet my need to be as near the front of the business we are going to as is possible. Yet, you would not believe how often I get comments from people who are angry because I am in a disabled spot. The most common complaint is since I have two good legs to walk on, why can't I park out in the parking lot somewhere like everybody else. They fail to understand one of the most dangerous places for me and my guide dog is "out there in the parking lot somewhere." The less distance we have to walk through a parking lot, the safer we are. Cars backing in and out without looking are extremely dangerous. In the summertime, when the pavement is so hot that prolonged contact with a dog's paws can burn them, it is essential that we be parked as close to our destination as is possible. Let me give the reader an example of just how important a disabled parking spot can be.

One of the businesses I frequent has a disabled parking spot completely around to the side of their main business entrance. Since there is no sidewalk much of the way down that side of the building, I and my guide dog have to walk behind a lot of cars. The problem is compounded because we frequent this business at night, making it much harder for any driver to see us. When I get out of the car, I have to navigate my way behind at least twenty to thirty cars to get to the front of the building where there is a sidewalk. One night, as I was making my way down the side of the building, a car suddenly began backing out as we walked behind it. Had I not yelled loudly and jumped out of the way with my guide dog, we would have been seriously injured when the driver backed over us. In fact, my dog would have probably been killed. On the nights the disabled parking spot is in use by a non disabled person, we have to park way out in the parking lot. Again, this requires my guide dog and I to travel behind upwards of one hundred cars. If we stop for every idling car, we would never get inside. Yet, passing behind these idling cars is not just dangerous. It is life threatening in the extreme. So, disabled people being so militant and vocal about their disabled parking spots is not without some justification.

You would not believe the times a disabled person cannot get into a disabled parking spot because a non disabled person is parked there. Here in the apartment complex I live in, we often come home to find the carpet cleaning truck in the disabled parking spot, or the pizza delivery person parked there, or non disabled neighbors. We often find the same situation at the local shopping center or mall. Please, if you are not disabled, do not use the disabled parking spots. It may seem like a minor infraction to you, but, to those who need those spots, it is a major inconvenience. Sometimes, it can be very dangerous for a disabled person to park anywhere else.

Again, you just never know when you will be the one with the disability. I went blind in my early forties due to a service connected disability I sustained while serving in the

Navy. As I said, Christopher Reeves became disabled in a riding accident in his late forties. It can happen to you. If you violate the rights of the disabled, and the blind, whether by parking in disabled parking spaces when you don't need to, or by denying people with service animals the exemptions afforded them by law, you are paving the way for people to discriminate against YOU if you ever become disabled. Help the disabled use and protect their rights now, just in case you need them yourself in the future.

Another sore spot for the disabled is the people who begrudge them for the stipends they receive from the government for their disabilities. My own relatives have always been extremely jealous and angry about the disability income I get from the Veteran's Administration. It is their opinion that I don't do anything for it. It is their opinion that it is grossly unfair for them to be working for a living while ***their*** taxes pay me a salary. They don't seem to have a clue to the fact I would gladly trade my situation for theirs in a heartbeat, not counting the fact that I have paid more than my fair share of taxes in my lifetime. If it were possible, I would gladly trade my blindness for their eyesight, their job for my disability income. I have talked to literally hundreds of other disabled people who get the same reaction from their relatives, resentment, anger, jealousy, and so on. What if these people had their way? What if we disabled people did not get these government stipends, as humble as most of them are. What if they suddenly found themselves disabled, unable to earn a living at their former career, or any career, and realized, that, thanks to people like them, disabled people no longer get disability stipends? Do you see where I am coming from? You never know when you will be the one who is disabled and in need of every right, and every disability benefit you can get.

The simple fact is, there is no need to begrudge disabled people for any income they may get from the state or federal government. I would rather be out riding motorcycles like I used to do than depend on others for my transportation. I would rather be out flying than trying to remember the feeling of soaring through the sky in my own airplane. I would much rather drive my own car than have to pay enormous taxi fees, or take an hour to get somewhere on a bus that would take ten minutes in a car. I know that other disabled and blind people share my sentiments in this regard. When I went to serve my country in the Navy, I did not join expecting to come home visually impaired and then to later go blind. But, I did. I can tell you, as a disabled veteran, I earned every single dime of every dollar the government will ever pay me. Just as any other disabled veteran has done. Again, be careful about begrudging the disabled their government stipends. Someday YOU may be disabled and have to depend on a government stipend too. Most disabled people would rather work and earn their own way if they can. Many disabled people do work full-time. Not only that, many of the disabled people who do not work full-time devote hundreds of hours a year to charitable causes and public service.

The blind have many other rights which most non disabled people take for granted everyday. Still, these are rights blind people are deprived of all the time. In December 1995 my wife and I went Christmas shopping at The Florida Mall in Orlando, Florida. One of the most basic right afforded to the blind is to have their guide dogs accompany them wherever they go. As a guide dog user, I was being accompanied by my guide dog, Frankie. I had just had my picture taken at a photo shop booth when I was approached by a cleaning lady. As I was handing the shop clerk the money for the picture this lady informed me I was to remove my guide dog from the mall property at once. I was amazed a mall would not know the laws pertaining to guide dogs. I was even more amazed a cleaning lady would be the one trying to challenge my right to have my guide dog with me at The Florida Mall.

I told the cleaning lady, as politely as I knew how, that my right to be accompanied in any public place by my guide dog was protected by Florida State law. She then rudely told me I would have to discuss the matter with a mall security officer. The cleaning lady left without another word. A few minutes later I heard someone walk up to me and step right in front of me. The person just stood there without saying a word to me. Finally, I asked who it was standing there because it was obvious they were not going to introduce who they were. As it turned out, it was a mall security officer. He gruffly asked me for my guide dog I.D. card to prove Frankie was a bona fide guide dog. I showed it to him and he walked away. No apology, no thanks for showing him the card, nothing on his part to show he regretted bothering me.

On another occasion my wife and I walked into a Winn-

Dixie store here in Orlando, Florida and were quickly met by a store manager. He was frantically trying to get to me before I got into the store with my guide dog. When he did get to me he told me to get out at once, that dogs were not allowed in the store. I went through my little talk about how guide dogs are guaranteed access by state and federal laws. At which point he let us in with some reservation. On still another occasion the same thing happened at a restaurant in St. Augustine, Florida.

The point of relating these incidents to the reader is to show how blind people are often denied the same rights non-disabled people take for granted. Which is why I maintain no one should ever begrudge a blind or disabled person for any right they have.

I have one more example of how blind people are often denied the most basic right. My wife and I were vacationing in West Yellowstone, Montana in September 1996 when I encountered a most distasteful example of discrimination. Along with a friend, my wife, guide dog, and I went walking into a local restaurant to eat lunch. When the waitress came to seat us she informed us we would have to sit in a back corner, away from the other diners. When I asked why we would have to be set apart from the rest of the customers she informed me they did not want dogs in their main dining area. If we wanted to eat in their establishment it would have to be in a back corner, away from the rest of the customers. We were all hungry, and I was not in the mood to argue guide dog access right then. So, we went in and ate our meal in a back corner, set apart from all the other customers. What the owner did not know is that his employee had just violated the American's With Disabilities Act, as well as Montana State law pertaining to guide dog access. If I had felt inclined to pursue the matter in Court the owner of this business could have wound up paying fines in excess of $50,000. Since I was not from the area I did not want to get tangled up in a legal situation which would require my return.

The crucial point is this. There is no reason to deny, or to begrudge the disabled their hard won rights. As I have stated many, many times in this book, you just never know when YOU might be a disabled person yourself, or have a son, or a daughter, or spouse that is disabled. Help protect the rights of the disabled.

FASCINATING FACTS ABOUT THE BLIND!

I typed this book on a computer. I was showing part of the manuscript to a friend one day to get their opinion on the content of one chapter. When they were done reading it, they asked me how I could see to do this. My friend had never seen my computer, and did not realize it talked or read me anything and everything displayed on the screen. So, I thought I would take this opportunity to explain how the blind can do some of the things not covered in the other chapters.

For example, I and my fellow blind friends ***listen*** to books and magazines. I get dozens of magazines on cassette tape and on records. These include Reader's Digest, Prevention, U.S. News & World Report, Outside, and many other popular magazines. I get talking books from the local library. Like many people, I like to read my local newspaper daily. Thanks to our local public broadcasting station, WMFE, I can ***listen*** to my local newspaper because dedicated volunteers at the station read the entire paper to all the blind people in our listening area every morning. Public Radio provides this service all over the United States. The stations even furnish the special radios required to pick up the broadcast. In fact, let me take this opportunity to thank all the selfless volunteers all over America who get up every morning and head down to their local public broadcasting station to read blind, visually impaired, and other print disabled people, their morning news. Unfortunately, we blind people enjoy these services, but, often forget to let the volunteers who make them possible know how much we appreciate them. In fact, just this morning, the WMFE Audio Reading Service volunteers made an announcement over the air that they would like to hear from blind listeners on how they liked the service. I took the time to call the number given in the announcement expecting to get a message machine. I got one of the volunteers helping read the newspaper that morning. So, I took the opportunity to say thank you to him and all the other volunteers for providing the reading service. He was bubbling over with happiness about getting to talk to one of the people he spent so much time and energy reading the paper for every morning. In talking with him it became clear they almost never heard from anyone they provided the service too. I hope, we as blind people, never forget many of the services we receive from the sighted community are not owed to us by anyone. Many of these volunteer services are provided by people who care about us as blind people. They deserve all the thanks and gratitude we can give them.

I am a coffee drinker, a habit I picked up during my Navy days. When I pour myself a cup of coffee, I use a special little device that sounds a little buzzer when my coffee reaches the top of the cup so I will not overfill it. I have another buzzer that sounds when I am filling the bathtub with water so I will not accidentally overfill it either.

Blind people can tell time with a braille watch they can either feel of, or listen to. We use talking scales which tell us our weight aloud since we cannot read a regular weight scale. In fact, I have great fun with my talking weight scale when friends come over to visit. Many a friend has taken the bait when I asked them to get on the scale and then had their weight announced aloud for all to hear. I have found it can be a dangerous thing to do with women friends.

When I have a book or magazine I want to read that I

cannot get on a tape cassette or on a record, I use a scanner to load it into my computer. Then, a special computer program I have, called Open Book, made by Arkenstone, reads the material back to me. That is how I go over my bank statement and my phone bill. I scan them into the computer, and then the computer reads them back to me.

My stove dial, my microwave dial, the washing machine dials are all marked in braille so I can be a nice husband and help my wife with the cooking and laundry. Boy, does she see to it that those braille dots stay in good shape, too. When one falls off, she puts it right back on.

When I eat a meal at home, or at a restaurant, I use a knife in one hand to locate my food, and then I grab it with my fork and down it goes. By spotting my food with my knife, I am able to eat without using my hands or fingers to locate my food. This is important for two reasons. One, the single biggest complaint sighted people have about blind people is they can be messy eaters. When I could see I was around many blind people who routinely ate their food with their hands and fingers. While one is tempted to make excuses for blind people who pick up their food with their fingers and eat like children, it would be an insult to blind people in general to do so. There is no excuse for a grown blind person eating like a baby, using their fingers to shovel their mashed potatoes, peas, and other food into their mouths. Finger food is a different matter, of course. Blind rehabilitation centers do train blind people how to eat properly, using their knife or another utensil to find their food and pick it up with a fork or spoon and eat properly. It is important for blind people to be well mannered when eating, at home, or in public. How a blind person eats in public affects how sighted people view all other blind people.

Another reason a blind person should use proper eating techniques is because it is easier than shoveling food into your mouth with your hands or fingers. I know a couple of legally blind people who can see their plates; but, the food on their plates is a blurry haze. To try to see their food better, they put their face down and in their plate about an inch above their food. Then, they shovel the food in without any regard to what it is they are eating. Others just mix up all their food into one big mess and eat it that way. The point is they spoil their own enjoyment of their meal for the sake of what might be an easier way to eat. If they took the time to get a little training, they could enjoy their meal sitting in an upright, more comfortable position. They could savor the flavor of the individual foods the way a person was meant to.

The list goes on. Blind people thread sewing needles with an automatic threader. I put safety pins in the hem of my pants in different positions so I can tell my pants apart. The blind put braille labels or other markers on prescription medicines to prevent accidentally taking the wrong medication or inadvertently take an overdose. I have a special ruler with engraved markings so I can accurately measure things too within 1/8". I tell time with a talking watch. I can find my way around town or hiking in the woods with a talking compass and braille maps. When my friends come over, we play braille Scrabble. There is a braille Monopoly game.

All these gadgets and electronic wonders do not solve all the problems blind people face, however. As a man, I can only imagine the difficulties blind women have in properly applying their makeup. I know they can learn how, and that putting on makeup properly is often one of the first concerns voiced by many women who go blind later in life. The little things that do not seem very important to a sighted person require some unique techniques if you are blind. For example, how do you know how much toothpaste is on your toothbrush if you cannot see it? A lot of blind people apply the toothpaste to their finger, and then put it on their toothbrush. How do you know you have your shirt or blouse on right side out if you are blind? Hey, even sighted people walk out of their house sometimes with their clothes on the wrong way. Well, a blind person feels of the tag to make sure it is on the inside where it belongs. How about something as basic as cleaning yourself after having a bowel movement? This may sound like to gross a subject to deal with, or highly inappropriate to talk about in a book like this. This item is a perfect example of what a blind person has to deal with all the time. Again, how would ***you*** determine you had cleaned yourself properly after a bowel movement if you were blind? Close your eyes and see what YOU would come up within that situation. Remember what senses you are working with, smell, touch, taste, and hearing.

Imagine you are out in public going somewhere with your cane and it breaks. Canes do get broken or bent. Since your cane would be the ***only*** way you could tell where you were, how would you get home or get the attention of a sighted person to help you?

Imagine yourself in this situation. You are out walking with your guide dog and he gets viciously attacked by another dog. All you know is your dog is in a fight for its life with another dog. You have no way to help your dog. If you kick out, you may injure your own dog. If you use pepper spray or maze, you may accidentally use it on your dog and wind up helping the other dog kill or severely injure your own guide dog. Well, I have had this experience happen to me; so have a lot of other blind people. Dealing with a similar situation would be hard, of course, for a sighted person out walking their pet. If you are blind, it is absolutely the most terrifying experience you can have.

Blind people deserve every ounce of respect and understanding a sighted person can muster. They have a special courage and dignity that deserves everyone's respect. There are blind people who languish in their apartments feeling sorry for themselves that is true. There are blind people who, through lack of training, cannot function well in public; but, the vast majority of blind people lead productive, normal lives. Blind mothers and fathers raise their children to be productive members of society. Blind lawyers argue eloquently on behalf of their clients before the court. Blind government workers prepare Social Security claims. Blind people function just as effectively as sighted people in almost every vocation that exists. Sure, they need special aids and training to cope with their blindness. If you ever want to get a hint of the courage and dignity all blind people deserve, get up one morning and blindfold yourself; see how much you can do and how well you can cope for a few hours.

Here is an interesting side note which illustrates something blind people do but sighted people don't think they can. Many states have pet laws that require pet owners to scoop up their pets droppings, or "poop." In almost every state with such laws, blind people are exempt. The reasoning is since a blind person cannot ***see*** where their dog pooped, they cannot pick it up. Therefore, they should not be required by law to do something they cannot do. Well, guess what? Guide dogs are trained at a number of guide dog schools to spin around in a circle just before they poop to alert their user he or she needs to be ready to pick up their droppings. The guide dog does not do this spin before urinating, only before dropping the poop. This allows a blind person the time to run their hand down the back of their dog so that it rests on the dog's back leg. The moment the dog is finished and steps away from the droppings the blind person can drop their free hand straight down to where the dog was voiding and pick up the droppings in a plastic bag. The poop can then be disposed of in a sanitary manner. You will find most guide dog users pick up after their guide dogs whether there is a law requiring them to do so or not.

I could go on and on about special devices for the blind. I can take my own blood pressure with a talking blood pressure monitor. When I do my aerobics, I can listen to my heart rate with a talking heart rate monitor. Don't get me wrong, as I said, all the answers to being blind are not found in electronics; but, the age of electronics has brought a lot of solutions to problems faced by blind people. The ingenuity of blind people will always take care of a lot of the things electronics don't.

GOD IS NOT THE CAUSE OF BLINDNESS!

I received many letters about this topic. In fact, I got a lot more letters about this than I would have ever expected to. I would have thought in our modern day society, people would not suffer under the delusion God is somehow responsible for blindness and punishes people by making them blind. Apparently I was wrong. I got a lot of letters from people tired of the notion that they are blind because God made them that way, or afflicted them for some grave wrong on their part. Because faith and religion are such sensitive subjects, I am not going to give the names of the people who wrote these letters, or print actual excerpts from them. Instead, I am going just to get to the heart of the matter, based on the content of the letters I got.

Blindness is just like any other affliction or disability. Blindness afflicts certain people, but not others. Lack of proper eye protection when using a tanning bed can cause permanent eye damage or blindness. If I do not use proper eye protection and suffer irreversible eye damage in a tanning bed that is not God's fault. If I run into a tree branch and poke out one of my eyes and become blind it was an accident that could have happened to anybody. It is not God's vindictive judgement on me for something I did wrong.

God does not go around afflicting people with blindness, or muscular dystrophy, or polio, or heart disease. We live in an imperfect world full of pain, suffering and disease, and while God allows bad things to happen to us, it does not mean that God makes these bad things happen to us. If you are a Christian, and you just have to blame someone for the bad things happening in life, blame the devil. I am a Christian; and from my study of the Bible, it is clear, while God allows bad things to happen to good people, like Job, God does not target people for things they have done wrong and then make them go blind. If He did, I have a funny feeling that blind people would not be a minority. The entire whole of humankind would have been struck blind because we all make mistakes. I know there are self righteous people out there who think they have never done anything wrong, or live perfectly before God in and of their own right, by their own works; but, everything I read in the Bible tells me we have all sinned and come short of the glory of God, to paraphrase Romans 3:23.

While we are on the subject of whether or not God blinds people out of some perverse sense of humor, let us take a quick look at another related topic I received hundreds of letters about the subject of healing. You would not believe the blind people who wrote to me to tell me about what they considered to be horrible experiences concerning attempted healings of their blindness by charismatic or other Christian healers. This is something I have even listened to on cable television.

I am old enough to remember an outstanding actor by the name of Clint Walker. He was a movie star for many years and starred in quite a few westerns. I was channel surfing one day and heard him talking and stopped to hear what he had to say. As it turned out, he was giving a personal testimony on a religious telecast on a Christian television station. His testimony was he loved God. Clint Walker, as it turned out, was losing his eyesight, and was apparently already legally blind. It was his hope and prayer on that day, in that Christian miracle crusade, God would fully restore his sight. Clint Walker, like every other sane person, did not want to lose his sight. Like many blind people, he turned to God for healing.

Needless to say, I stayed tuned to the broadcast to hear what finally happened to Clint Walker in that healing crusade. Since the evangelist was, and still is, a healer of some renown, I wanted to see just what he could do for a blind or visually impaired person. The evangelist said the words, he slapped Clint Walker on the forehead and yelled, "Be healed." Nothing happened. There was no change in Clint Walker's vision. A frustrated evangelist went on to explain it was not he; but God who provided the healing, and any healing was totally dependent on the faith of the person requesting the healing. A very emotional Clint Walker left the stage not knowing if, or when, any healing would be forthcoming. To my knowledge no healing ever occurred. In fairness to the evangelist, and to Clint Walker, I do not believe it was any reflection on either one of them that Clint Walker was not healed. God allows disabled people to remain in the world, in my opinion, to teach the rest of humanity how to be kind and tolerant of others, and to teach the people so afflicted to learn to trust and depend on Him for their help and salvation.

The reason I bring this episode to the sighted reader is because it is a perfect example of what many disabled people go through at the hands of people who claim to be healers, evangelist, or vehicles for God's healing power. Disabled people frequently get talked into going to healing crusades by religious friends or relatives on the pretense, if they just have enough faith, they will come home sighted, or walking, or hearing, or whatever it is they need to be made whole. Clint Walker wound up having the same experience many disabled people have had at these healing crusades. They go home just as blind, or just as deaf, or just as crippled as when they walked in the door. In Clint Walker's case, it was especially sad because it was very clear the evangelist was making full use of the fact a celebrity had come to him, above all others, for a healing miracle. The evangelist got the benefit of the celebrity of Mr. Walker without ever giving him anything in return, namely his vision.

I cannot tell you how many blind and disabled people I have talked too over the years who were told the only reason God did not heal them was because their life was not right, or they did not have enough faith, or they belonged to the wrong church, or they should have spoken in tongues. As I said in the last paragraph, I believe very strongly if God, in His Infinite Wisdom, chooses to heal a person, that person will be healed of their affliction, whatever that affliction happens to be. I also believe very strongly God allows many of us to remain afflicted because it somehow enriches not only our lives, but the lives of all we come into contact with. God is more than able to meet the needs of any disabled person, and in my opinion, all disabled people have the assurance in the Bible when God resurrects us at His Second Coming we will all have perfect bodies.

In the meantime, the blind and other disabled people should not be made to feel spiritually inferior if God does not heal them at a miracle crusade or church meeting. If a blind person wants to go to such a meeting to seek a healing, I fully agree that he should go. I do believe if God chooses, He can heal them. It is terribly wrong for sighted Christians who fail to heal a blind person, or a deaf person, to blame the disabled person for the lack of healing, or to even assume that blind or disabled people attending their services are there to be healed.

I was at such a service one time and had an incident occur which I think illustrates my last statement. I went with a friend, at the friend's invitation. Since their method of worship was different from what I was accustomed to, I sat quietly throughout the service, even though the main congregation was quite energetic. I enjoyed this energy, but in my own way. Well, at the end of the service a gentleman walked up to me and palmed a slip of paper into my hand and told me to have someone read it to me when I got home. When I got home, I did have someone read it to me. As it turned out, the slip of paper contained a long line of scripture references the man wanted me to hear. When my friend read me these scripture references, it became clear; because I had not gone forward to be healed during the healing service that followed the worship service, this man had judged me to be unsaved, a nonbeliever, in danger of hellfire, and one who rejected the healing power of God as a heathen of the worst order. I guess it never occurred to him not every disabled person who comes to their church comes there for healing. I know disabled people who do not go to church specifically because of attitudes like the one this man displayed toward me.

Again, one need only look at the life of Helen Keller to realize the blessing a disabled person can bring to the world. Louis Braille would have never brought the reading and writing system of braille to millions of blind people down through the centuries if he had not become blind himself. I hope sighted people will realize it is no sin to be blind, or otherwise disabled. The blind and disabled make great contributions to society that a sighted person might not make.

I cannot think of a better note to end this chapter on than Revelation 1:7. In it God promises, "Behold, he cometh in clouds, ***and every eye shall see him...***" That is the day all blind people will see.

DO SOMETHING KIND FOR A BLIND PERSON YOU MEET TODAY!

I made the statement in the Introduction to this book that it was not going to be the vehicle for whining blind people; and, I am going to stick by that statement. There are times when those who are fortunate enough not to be disabled could make the lives of the blind and disabled a little easier to deal with. Most blind and disabled people are very independent. So, the last thing we want is for people to be making life easier for us just to make it easier for us. That may sound like a confusing statement. What it means is this. For the most part, the blind and the disabled can take care of themselves. We do not need sighted people trying to help us in ways we do not need the help, as I pointed out in various parts of this book. It never hurts to ask if we need help; I pointed that out too. There are times, however, when a random act of kindness to a blind or disabled person can really make our day easier.

Let me give you an example. I just moved into a new apartment complex, a very large complex in fact. I am still learning my way around it with my guide dog, Frankie. One of the routes we have had to learn is how to get to the mailbox. In a few days, or in a week or two, getting to the mailbox will be a piece of cake. But, since we have only been here a day or two, it is still quite a challenge. Well, Frankie and I just made the circuitous route to the central mail point for our part of the apartment complex. This is one of those mail points where there are maybe fifty or sixty boxes, and there is usually a crowd of people elbowing each other to get to their mail. When we got there, I told Frankie to head for our corner. From this corner I am able to find the bottom of the boxes and then count more than six mail box locks to our box. Our box is the sixth lock over. I immediately realized all the doors were open, and the mail carrier was still putting out the mail. However, I had no idea how long he would be, so I asked him. All he would tell me was he was not done yet. Well, that was obvious enough already. All I needed to know from him was how much longer he would be. I did not want to walk back to our apartment if he would be done in a minute or two. Nor, did

I want to stay if he were going to be another fifteen or twenty minutes. The mail carrier would not tell me. Frankie and I turned around to head out of the mail center. Since all the main doors were apparently open and blocking our exit, Frankie did not want to proceed. Some assistance would have clearly been helpful at this point. If the mail carrier had closed one or two of the doors blocking our path, we could have exited more easily. He wouldn't help in that regard either. Finally, I got Frankie to thread our way past these doors and off toward home.

Let me suggest how a random act of kindness at this point could have really made a difference. Because a blind man with a guide dog had made his way, from who knows where, it should have occurred to this mail man that it was with some difficulty that we got there at all. He could have asked for me to show him my key to verify I really lived there and then handed me my mail so I would not have to make a return trip. Total interruption time to him would have been a few minutes at the most. We would have had our mail, and been home with no need to return. While I normally expect no help whatever with my mail, on this particular day, being new to the complex and the route to the mailbox, such an act of kindness would have been deeply appreciated.

Let me give the reader another example. My wife and I shop at a particular grocery store in Orlando, Florida. We have been shopping in the same store for years. The store has a policy for the bag persons, or whatever they are called now, always to ask the customer if they need assistance out with their groceries after they have paid for them. My wife and I appreciate this because she has a bad back, and I am busy navigating my way through doors and around obstacles with my guide dog. Now, I suppose I could take the front of the cart like I do inside the grocery store and pull it out with my guide dog's help. The point is this, the bag persons frequently do not bother following the store policy to ask if we need assistance out with our groceries. It seems obvious to me, if they were going to forget to ask someone this question, a blind or disabled person would be the last person they would forget to offer this help too. Here is an excellent example of how a random act of kindness would really make the day of a blind person. As I pointed out, in this case, it is store policy to ask.

It is true that these two examples were from my personal

experiences. I have gotten literally hundreds of letters saying the same thing. Again, blind and disabled people do not expect to be pampered or waited on hand and foot by the public. There are times when a random act of kindness would really help us. The times these are needed are usually so obvious it is hard to understand why sighted people have a hard time figuring out that some act of kindness would help in certain situations.

To close this chapter on a positive note, let me give an example of two "random" acts of kindness for a disabled person. I had another mail carrier I dealt with that exemplifies the manner in which sighted people can show kindness to the blind or disabled. When our mail carrier has mail for people in our apartment, but the items are too large for our regular mailbox, he puts them in a larger box and leaves the key to this larger box in our regular mailbox. The problem for a blind person is, when you find a key in your mailbox, you have no way of knowing which of ten larger boxes it belongs to. If there are no fellow residents around to ask which box the key goes to, a blind resident cannot retrieve his or her other mail. Well, I had a mail carrier come along one day who noticed I was unable to use the key without someone telling me which box it went to. He then told me he would always put my mail in a certain box which was on the corner and very easy to locate by feel. Anytime I found a key in my mailbox I automatically would know it went to this box. All I had to do was locate this box and retrieve my additional mail. The plan worked like a charm. It turned what had been a real problem into a practical solution. Yet, this was something the mail carrier did not have to do. It was a random act of kindness.

It does not hurt for blind people to do a few acts of kindness for other blind people, or the sighted, or other disabled people whenever possible. Being blind does not mean that we cannot donate our time and energies to community projects just like the sighted do. I, and a number of other blind people in my area also write, publish, and distribute brochures that help explain how to serve blind customers when they shop in a business, or how better to relate to a guide dog team when you encounter one. In fact, I have written a booklet called "You Have A New Neighbor" that new guide dog users can send out, or hand out to their neighbors, that educates them on guide dog teams. I know of other blind people who regularly go to the blood bank and donate blood. Other blind people I know give free lectures and seminars at schools and civic clubs on what it is like to be blind and how blind people are productive members of the community. Many of these blind people do these activities in addition to holding down regular jobs and while managing families and households.

TIPS ON BEING A SIGHTED SPOUSE!

I got a surprising amount of mail from blind people on this subject. It was a total surprise to me. I simply did not expect the sighted spouses of blind people to need tips on how to help their blind "better halves" cope with their blindness. I knew I had encountered serious problems with my sighted spouse; but, I was surprised to learn the problem was widespread throughout the blind community.

The problem is this. Blind and visually impaired people undergo a lot of training to learn how to cope with their blindness; but, our spouses almost never undergo any training on how to be a better sighted spouse. This is surprising when you realize that one's spouse needs to know how and why blind people do things as much as blind people themselves do. For example, I came home with my guide dog after thirty days of very intense training. I knew how to get out of the car and safely go from the car to a curb, listen for oncoming traffic, and cross to another curb.

check the curb for height, and then, step onto the curb with my guide dog. When I got home and my wife and I went to the grocery store for the first time, I confidently got out of the car and proceeded very carefully to follow my training to get out of the parking lot and into the store. I had briefly explained to my wife what I would be doing. From the moment we left the car until we got into the store everything went wrong. My wife went out across the parking lot without any regard to the oncoming traffic. Instead of stopping at the curb so I could determine the flow of traffic, she just went barreling out into the lane of traffic assuming we had plenty of time to cross safely. Since I had told my guide dog to follow her, he was confused about whether to do what they trained us to do, or try to keep up with my wife even though she was violating every rule we followed. This scene repeated itself dozens of times over the next year while I tried to teach my wife how to travel with me and my guide dog so we could follow the rules we had learned.

The point here is not to bash my wife. The fact is that no one had trained her intensely for thirty days on how to travel with a guide dog and blind spouse. No one had trained her on how to travel with a blind spouse using a cane. In fact, she had not been trained in any way, shape, form or fashion on how to be a sighted spouse. Since blind people are supposed to be totally self sufficient and independent I think the powers that be figure there is no reason to help a sighted spouse understand how to assist or work with a blind spouse. The result of this lack of training for sighted spouses is there is a lot of friction in marriages. Many blind spouses are always at odds with their sighted spouse because the sighted spouse doesn't know how blind people do things. It seems incredible that a sighted spouse would not take the time to learn the things he or she needs to know better to work with a blind spouse. But where is the sighted spouse supposed to get the proper information to cope with their blind spouse more effectively and efficiently? Usually, the only source for this information is the blind spouse. It is no secret that blind spouses are not always the best teachers.

There is no doubt there should be some form of in home training for sighted spouses to parallel the training their blind spouse gets. If there is such training in use somewhere today, it is a total mystery to thousands of blind couples. In my checks with a number of blind service agencies, no one could tell me of such a program. So, here are some tips for sighted spouses on how they can better assist their blind partners.

It is critical that things remain constant in the home of a blind person. My wife used to make major changes in our home every month or two. I would then spend weeks relearning the layout of the furniture, cabinet contents, what have you. About the time I got the new layout down, she would change it all again. I finally got her to stop doing this. From the mail I got, this is apparently a very common problem. This does not mean you cannot change the layout of your home occasionally. Such changes should not occur more than once or twice a year.

Another important tip is that a sighted spouse should learn to travel, or walk, using the very same techniques their blind partner uses. If your blind partner uses a guide dog; then, as a sighted spouse, you ought to follow the same rules of mobility your blind partner uses with their guide dog. No cutting across parking lots, no passing up curb corners to make a quick crossing, just because, you can see no cars are coming. When I first came home with my guide dog, Frankie, my wife would go darting out into traffic and between cars because she thought she had enough room to get through. She would be all the way across the parking lot lane while my guide dog and I would still be across the lane, at the curb, trying to figure out the traffic flow. We were often trying to figure out where my wife was. Had we followed her, my guide dog would have unlearned his training and begun to do things the wrong way. The only proper solution was for my wife to learn to travel the way we needed to. But, I was the one who had gone to guide dog school and had the thirty days of intense training, not my wife. It is my sincere opinion every guide dog school and blind rehab center ought to include a week of training with the sighted spouse AND the blind client. Then, when the blind client gets back home the sighted spouse knows what to do to help their blind partner use their training. The sighted spouse will have then learned what to do, firsthand from the professionals. We hope they will have trained the sighted spouse with a blindfold so they know just how stressful traveling blind can be; and, how critical it is for those traveling with a blind person to observe the same travel rules their blind partner has to observe.

Another important point for a sighted spouse to keep in mind is this. Never just walk away from your blind partner without telling them you have done so. The reader will no doubt notice that this is a tip I have already mentioned in a previous chapter; and, it is a tip that a sighted spouse, of all people, should know to follow. Unfortunately, this is something many sighted spouses do all the time. They just walk away from their blind partner and leave them standing there, like a tree in the middle of a pasture. As a result, the blind spouse has no one to talk to. They have no idea where their sighted spouse has gone, or when they will be back. Believe me, when I tell you, a few minutes of standing alone in the middle of a store seem like an eternity to a blind person. A friend might not know better; but, a sighted spouse should know not to leave their blind spouse standing alone without telling them they are stepping away for a few minutes. In fact, this reminds me of an occasion when my wife and I were in the local Wal-Mart store. I had not heard a peep out of my wife for about five minutes. Since we had apparently gotten in a long line, I assumed we were just not moving along. Then someone next to me was asking me if I were lost. I replied, "No," and told them I was waiting in line with my wife. This kind person told me I was standing at least fifteen feet away from the register, right out in the middle of the floor, and there was no wife near me. Further, she informed me, I had been standing there alone for at least ten minutes. She was afraid I was lost and just did not know what to do. About that time, my wife overheard the conversation and came back to me telling me she had not noticed I was not with her. Not only was I soundly humiliated, but the shopper who was kind enough to come to my aid was flabbergasted that a sighted spouse could not notice her blind husband was not with her.

Here is another tip. Tell your blind spouse if there is enough clearance to open his or her car door when getting out of the car. I find I have to ask frequently if I have enough clearance to open my car door when my wife and I go somewhere. I do not want to open the door and bang the door into someone's car. First, I do not want to damage their car and have to pay for a paint job; and two, I do not want to damage our car and have to pay for a paint job. I got a number of letters on this tip. One lady wrote to tell me that despite years of begging her husband to tell her if she had clearance to open her car door, he continued to insist that she ask. Her attitude was that he knew she was going to have to know every single time. Therefore, he knew to tell her whether she asked or not. His stubborn insistence on making her ask every single time was a really sore point in their relationship. As a common courtesy, she felt that her sighted spouse should have told her without her having to ask. Something like this might seem like a trivial thing to most sighted people; but, to a blind person, such incidents are an indication that their blindness is a burden to those around them. It is felt their blindness makes them somehow unworthy of special considerations that would go a long way toward making their daily life easier. When such inconsiderate behavior comes from a sighted spouse, the feelings of being a burden or somehow unworthy is magnified tenfold.

I want to be sure the sighted reader does not misunderstand the intent of this chapter. Any blind person knows it can be a burden to a spouse, a friend, or to relatives, to have a blind person in their midst. There is absolutely no doubt that traveling with, or living with, a blind person requires the sighted partner, friend, or relative to do things differently than they would if they were not with a blind person. The point is this. If you as a sighted spouse, or friend, or relative were blind, you would want the same courtesies, the same benefits, and the same help any other blind person does now. You just cannot imagine how some of the smallest courtesies can make a huge difference in the lives of blind people you know. That is all this chapter is trying to point out. If you are the sighted spouse of a blind person, your blind spouse is fully aware of the problems their blindness poses for you. While I know blind people can be demanding at times, blindness itself is also extremely demanding at times. It requires 100% of a blind person's energies to cope with their blindness every moment of every single day. If you, as a sighted spouse, can help your blind partner have a better day through the extending of little courtesies, or following their method of traveling or coping with things, then do it. Someday you might just find yourself walking in the shoes of a blind person, and then you will expect all the same courtesies and help.

There are hundreds of other little tips that sighted spouses should know about. While I cannot cover them all in a book of this length, here are a few more notable tips that will help any sighted spouse in dealing with their partner's blindness.

Do not speak for your spouse in a conversation. Let your

spouse speak for themselves. It is common for sighted people to talk among themselves and totally ignore a blind person who is standing right there who, if sighted, would be included in the conversation without any question. Sighted spouses often find it easier to speak for their blind partner rather than letting the blind partner in on the conversation. Again, include your blind partner in the conversation. If the sighted person you are talking to continues to ask you questions that should be directed to your blind spouse, tell the sighted person to ask your blind spouse as he or she would be the better person to answer that particular question.

Fill your blind spouse in on what is happening when you are out and about. For example, my wife and I will go to pick out a Hallmark card for some friend or relative for a special occasion. I will often hear my wife thumbing through card after card without saying a word to me. Finally, I will ask her to describe the cards she is looking at to me so I can help decide what card we will buy. Other blind people have told me that when they go to buy shoes or clothes that their sighted spouse will discuss colors and styles of clothes with the sales person, but never ask them if this is something they would like to buy or wear. Remember, blind people are fully aware of what they like and don't like. Include your blind spouse in making clothing or other choices when out shopping.

Here is a tip I got a lot of mail on. Without pampering your blind spouse like a child, give them the once over before you go somewhere like to church. I have actually had people walk up to me at church to tell me I had some glaring pieces of lint on my suit coat. Sometime it will be something like a shirt collar turned up in back, or a pant leg so wrinkled I should have never walked out of the house wearing those particular pants. Many of the letters I received on this subject related similar tales of embarrassing situations that could have been avoided if their spouse had just glanced at their clothes and overall appearance before they left home. As independent as blind people are, as good as we are about dressing and grooming, we can make mistakes. Mistakes that we do not spot because we are blind. Mistakes that a sighted person would have caught in a mirror. I would much rather have my spouse give me the once over before we leave home, than to have a sighted friend come up to me in church or a restaurant to tell me that I have a big piece of dryer lint hanging from the lapel of my suit coat.

Lest sighted spouses who read this book think that they are unappreciated, let me close this section on a positive note. Being the spouse of a blind person is a lot like being blind. A sighted spouse has to arrange things in certain ways in the kitchen to make it easier for their blind spouse to get to what they need. A sighted spouse has to live with food cans with braille labels on them. They have to remember to tell us where the food is on our plates. They have to put up with taking us where we need to go when a bus or a taxi will not do. Sighted spouses never know what we think about their new hairdo or haircut, because we cannot see it. When my wife wants to know how she looks in a new outfit, I cannot tell her because I cannot see it. No matter how pretty she makes herself for me, I have no way of knowing unless she tells me and then describes herself to me. If she loses weight, I will not notice. The list goes on. There is no doubt about it; sighted spouses deserve an extra word of praise for the often selfless dedication they show to their blind or visually impaired partners. This is not to say that blind spouses are a burden to their sighted partners. I do not want a lot of angry letters coming in from blind readers who think I am suggesting that blind spouses are a burden. All I am saying is sighted spouses do go the extra mile for we blind spouses occasionally. We would show the most arrogant ingratitude to believe otherwise.

There is, of course, the positive side to being married to a blind spouse. When my wife takes me to the beach, I cannot see the bikini clad women. I cannot see her looking at and drooling over the handsome European men. My wife can dress me funnily and I might not realize it in time to change into something different. I don't get excited about cute waitresses when we eat out. She can run through yellow lights at intersections without me knowing it.

A BLIND PERSON'S VISION FOR THE FUTURE!

Blind people often listen to every news bulletin about some new technological development for the blind. Just the other night, I, and thousands of other blind people, listened with that same bated breath as a news piece on DATELINE on NBC told about a new device which I mentioned earlier in this book. This is the device called Strider that allows blind people to use a satellite locating system to travel about in their community and always know where they are. When we heard the going price would be $4000, we all gasped a sigh of disappointment realizing that this system, like so many others, would be out of our reach.

Most blind people depend on the government, or charitable civic groups, or non profit foundations for the blind, to provide such expensive equipment to them because most of us cannot simply afford to spend that kind of money. Even a blind person, who works full time and makes a good living, cannot afford such equipment. The problem is that many of these service providers, the government in particular, do very little to provide this kind of technology to the blind. There are no plans available that allow a blind person to get and be using this type of new technology while they pay for it on a time payment plan.

I have been extremely fortunate in that I am a disabled Navy veteran whose blindness is the result of my military service. As a service connected, disabled veteran, the Veteran's Administration has helped me get some of the equipment I need. Even then, the waiting list for such equipment can be up to two years. Further, the government, whether it is the Social Security Administration or the Veteran's Administration, does not make much of the better technology available to the blind. For example, I do not know of any program available to any blind person at present that allows them to get the new Strider mobility location system at no cost, or on a payment plan. This is important to blind people on a fixed income who need help to get the system. Computer technology is another good example of how blind people cannot frequently get technology that would greatly enhance their daily lives.

I have a talking computer equipped with a scanner which

allows me to scan printed material into my computer and then have the computer read it back to me. The computer also talks to me and reads me anything displayed on the screen in my Windows program. Since I am an author I donate a considerable amount of desktop publishing work to charities. This computer was critical to my being able to do my work. I also needed my computer to scan in printed material like my mail, my bills, and other items I needed my computer to read to me. Now, if I had wanted to wait one to two years, the V.A. would have probably bought this computer system for me. I did not have one to two years to wait. Think about it. Can you imagine sitting around your house day after day, week after week, month after month, waiting for a computer system to be able to put in a productive day of work? What I did was use my own money to buy the system myself, money my wife and I really needed to buy a new car and pay bills with. Most blind people could not come up with the $6,000 I had to spend on my system at all. Which means most blind people in the community do not have access to a computer system that would act as a reading machine, and allow them to type letters and do other word processing on a computer that will read it back to them.

One thing blind people would desperately like to see is the government making as much modern technology available to them as possible, as soon as possible. Sighted people may argue this is just another example of the disabled expecting the sighted, or non disabled community, to subsidize their needs. Many blind people would argue this claim on my part just further demeans the blind by expecting charity from the sighted world. My feeling is if we can send billions of dollars to Russia we can provide this equipment to the disabled. If we can continue to dish out criminally high overpayments to those frauding Medicare we can give talking computers to the blind. If our government can continue to lend trillions of dollars to third world countries who hate America, then it can provide critically needed technology to the blind and visually impaired who will never have it otherwise.

Another thing a lot of blind people I talked to would like to see in the future is something I mentioned in a previous chapter, which is the widespread availability of large cell braille materials so older blind people, or blind people with finger sensitivity problems, can learn braille and use it in a form they can read. When I researched the availability of large cell braille, I was so shocked at the lack of availability of large cell braille that I was tempted to found an organization devoted to that purpose myself. I did not because I felt someone had to already be working to make such an important and critical resource available to the blind. As of this writing, the problem remains. Probably, because service providers feel with the availability of materials on audio tape, large cell braille would be redundant. Excuse me! We do not expect sighted people to use audio tapes in place of large print. So, why do we expect the blind to use audio tapes in place of large cell braille, the equivalent of large print for the sighted? I find it extremely interesting there is a form of braille called micro braille, a smaller version of standard braille for those with extremely sensitive fingers. The advantage to micro braille is that it saves space. It takes up less room than standard dot braille. Well, if we can have micro braille as an alternative; we should have large braille too.

Again, as I mentioned in an earlier chapter, less than 10% of all blind people know how to read braille. I discussed the reasons with a number of organizations that deal with the blind; not one could give a reason for this low number. In talking with a number of adult blind people, I came away with the simple conclusion that since the majority of blind people are older and have sensitivity problems they cannot read standard dot braille, but they can read large cell braille. The reason they do not pursue braille as an alternative is that, even if they learn braille, large cell braille, there are almost no materials available in large cell braille for them to use. In other words, why learn the only braille you can read, large cell braille, only to find there is very little in large cell braille to read. I also believe when all braille materials available in standard dot braille are also available in large cell braille, then the per centage of blind people who can read braille will skyrocket to 70% to 80%. Although, after years of large cell braille not being widely available, I do believe it will take a charitable organization devoted to teaching large cell braille and making it widely available to the blind public to make such a high per centage of braille readers a reality.

Another thing the blind would like to see is more public awareness in the business community about how to deal with the blind. I got hundreds of letters on this subject and have dealt with some of these issues in other parts of this book. Here are some aspects to the issue I have not dealt with which are very important to the blind.

I take my wife out to eat about once a week. Since we enjoy many foods, we often go to a different restaurant every week for months at a time. In the last year, I have had only two waitresses provide me with a braille menu. I have only encountered one waitress who knew how to set my food down and then tell me where she had set it. Every waitress and waiter in America ought to know exactly how to deal with a blind customer. It is part of the vision of the blind that someday all businesses will routinely train their staff on how to better serve the blind.

Let me give you another example. I have had people stop me at the door to restaurants to tell me dogs are not allowed in eating establishments. I finally got in, but, only after showing my little book of Access Laws for service animals and guide dogs. It is fair for restaurant staff to ask if my dog is trained to be in public places as a legitimate guide dog; but, that was not the issue. These people did not have a clue to the fact that such a thing as a guide dog or service animal even existed, or that they would allow such animals in a restaurant. I, and others I know, have been asked to leave shopping malls with our guide dogs.

There are businesses that market services to such businesses that instruct employees how on to deal with the blind. While I do not object to anyone making a profit, I would certainly like to see a charity established that would make it their primary objective to educate all businesses with regard to these matters. I have even thought of founding such a charity, because, it is something that needs to be done. After extensive research on whether or not such an organization existed, I could not find a single one that would go to businesses at no cost, or a nominal cost, to educate their staff about how to deal with the blind. While I am sure there must be some organization out there that includes this type of public education in its goal, there is much work left to be done. There is no reason such an organization could not be founded and administered by the blind.

No doubt, the future of the blind and disabled is in the hands of the blind and disabled. It is my hope this book has helped bring a better understanding about the blind to the sighted community. As I said in the Introduction, this book was never intended to be a brilliant dissertation or a literary masterpiece. I intended it to provide an easy read for sighted people. To provide practical information about how to relate to the blind and visually impaired. To give the blind some insight on ways we could help improve our relations with both the sighted community, and with our blind brothers and sisters.

I wish more blind people had responded to my request for their ideas for this book. To the hundreds of blind people that did respond, thank you. Your ideas helped make this book a valuable source of information and an educational tool to the community.

To service provider's and blind rehab specialists who read this book, remember, I am not trying to reach the professional field in this book. I am trying to reach the average person in the community who does not know very much about the blind and to whom this book is very informative and enlightening. I do hope it is well received for what it is within the professional community. Remember, the average person on the street doesn't know very much about the blind or disabled.

To the sighted people who read this book, I want to say the heartiest thank you of all. Unless this book gets read by sighted people, it will not be able to educate and inform the sighted world about what it is like to be blind. I hope copies of this book find their way into every school, college, library, church, rehab center, business establishment, and book store in America. I hope blind people care enough about educating their sighted friends and relatives to give this book to them as a gift. If you are sighted, and cared enough about the blind to read this book, you are to be highly commended. If you put the information you gleaned from this book to use, then you are to be even more highly commended.

I especially hope this book finds its way into every classroom in America. Why? Because, it is our children who hold the greatest promise of helping the sighted community deal more equitably with the blind. The technologies of the future that help the blind are probably going to be invented by the young people passing through our public and private schools right now. I hope teachers will encourage their students to get involved in working with the blind. In fact, one project I highly recommend as a school project, is the sponsoring of a guide dog for a blind person. This is an ambitious project since it can cost more than

$4000 to sponsor a guide dog.

The reason this particular project is so exciting is because your class gets to name the guide dog, and is kept updated on how the dog is doing in training, and who gets the dog when it goes out to do its work. The class would also get a picture of the dog and the blind person getting it when both graduate from guide dog school. Again, this is a very ambitious project for a school class to undertake. It is a project that benefits a blind person for many years. It is something every single participant in the class can be enormously proud of. If this is a project your class or civic club might want to consider, I have included a list of guide dog schools at the end of this book you can contact for more information on their sponsorship programs.

I would also like to recommend to local churches and civic groups around the country who have never done a project for the blind to do the same thing, sponsor a guide dog, or a talking computer system for a blind person in your own community. Unfortunately, not every blind person is eligible for help from the government with such systems. The only way some blind people will ever get them is if some church or civic group sponsors the devices for them.

While a talking computer, or a mobility device like the Strider, can be too costly for the average blind person to buy, it can be affordable to a church when all the members participate in a bake sale, or a special offering to raise the money to buy it. Here is a project I recommended to one church that they found very educational. Invite your congregation to bring blindfolds with them to a service. See what it is like to not be able to see the church hymnals during song service, or the offering plate when it is passed, or see the Pastor when he or she is giving the message.

I would like to recommend a project to the families and friends of blind and visually impaired people, too. Try being blind for half a day. Do it safely, but let yourself, with the proper supervision, be blind for a day, or part of a day. You will learn something of the courage and dignity required to cope with blindness. It will definitely give you a greater appreciation for the coping skills of your blind or visually impaired friends or relatives. (See Chapter One for suggestions on how to be blind for a few hours).

Another project that any business, church, school or a civic group can undertake is this. Look within your own facilities and see if you have braille signs and markers for the blind on the restroom doors. Are the classroom doors marked in braille? Usually such signs will not be up yet because your facility may not have any blind people accessing it. You never know when you will, so put them up as a class project. The cost to do so is minimal, and such signs are available at most office supply houses through their catalog.

Here is one last project for everyone. Give someone you know a copy of this book as a special gift. This sounds very self serving, I know, because it sounds like I am just trying to promote my book. However, a lot of sighted people will never pick up this book and read it unless someone who has read it gives it to them.

Let me leave one last thought with you. The blind may not be able to see physically, but the blind often sense a lot more than sighted people do because we make such full use of our remaining senses. Blind people deserve your respect and admiration, not your pity. Remember, you could well be blind or visually impaired yourself someday, or have a child or loved one who is blind or visually impaired. How you, as a sighted person, treat the blind and disabled today is going to determine how society treats you, or your loved one, should you ever go blind or become visually impaired in the future.

THE END

Additional print or audio cassette copies of this book may be obtained by sending $14.95, and $3.00 S&H, per copy to:

Harry Martin
2314 River Park Circle, #2111
Orlando, Florida 32817-4828

*** All checks should be made payable to Harry Martin. Please allow four weeks for delivery. Please specify print or audio.**

Civic clubs, church groups, and other organizations can purchase additional copies of this book in quantities of ten or more for $10.95, and $3.00 S&H, per copy. Quantities of fifty or more are $8.95, and $2.00 S&H per copy.

Harry Martin is available for speaking engagements on the subject matter presented in this book for a nominal fee. He is also available for two hour seminars to help businesses educate their staffs on how to better serve their blind and visually impaired customers. You may request available dates and fees by faxing your request to 407-382-1594, or by mailing your request to the address above.

ABOUT THE AUTHOR!

Harry Martin is a 100% Service-Connected disabled veteran who became disabled while serving in the Navy. Mr. Martin is a member of the Blinded Veteran's Association, a Life Member of Disabled American Veteran's, and a member of the American Legion.

Harry Martin is also the author of "What A Friend We Have In Jesus". Other informational booklets by Harry Martin include "You Have A New Neighbor" - There Is A Guide Dog In Your Neighborhood". This booklet helps new guide dog user's introduce their guide dogs to their neighbors.

Mr. Martin is an avid outdoors man whose interest's include backpacking, hiking, canoeing, and recreational walking. His wife, Carol, and his guide dog, Frankie, accompany him on his outdoor excursions. Harry also bowls on his churches bowling league.

In addition to his writing, and recreational interests, Harry lectures on the topic of this book, "WHAT BLIND

PEOPLE WISH SIGHTED PEOPLE KNEW ABOUT BLINDNESS."

Harry lives in Orlando, Florida with his wife and guide dog, Frankie, and often volunteers his time and resources to work as a volunteer advocate for the blind.

Since the original edition of this book was published in 1996 Harry Martin has become totally blind.

PROJECT RESOURCE LIST:

Guide Dog Schools...

Guiding Eyes for the Blind
611 Granite Springs Road
Yorktown Heights, NY 10598
914-245-4024

Leader Dogs for the Blind
1039 S. Rochester Road
Rochester, Michigan 48063
313-651-9011

Pilot Dogs, Inc.
625 West Town Street
Columbus, Ohio 43215
614-221-6367

Southeastern Guide Dogs
4210 77th Street East
Palmetto, Florida 33561
813-729-5665

OUTA SIGHT PRODUCTS

505 S. Beverly Drive, $438
Beverly Hills, CA 90212
Telephone: 1-800-246-5946
http://www.outasight.com

OUTA SIGHT PRODUCTS is a catalog company owned and operated by the blind. Outa Sight Products has just announced a new product line that has generated a tremendous amount of excitement throughout the blind community.

New Tagging System

Clothing tags with newly developed washer/dryer proof tape. Finally, a way to tag your clothing any way you wish. Make the label using a slate. Then, slide the tape into our tag holder and sew the soft, flexible tag into your clothes. Do it once and it will last as long as your clothes. The Braille will never disappear.

Totally reusable tags for everything else you can imagine. Can be used repeatedly. You can label whatever you want. However, you want, with any labeler. You can use these labels on everything from small bottles to large boxes of soap. You can even label items going into the freezer and the label won't ever come off.

New Electric Wall Plug Guide

A new wall plug cover that guides any plug into the wall socket. Impossible to make a mistake. No more getting shocked or frustrated because you can't find the wall plug - the special plug guide makes it simple. Easily fits over any wall socket in your home. Never before available.